52 PREPPER'S PROJECTS FOR PARENTS AND KIDS

A Project a Week to Help Prepare Your Child for the Unpredictable

David Nash

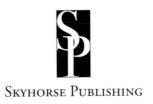

Skyhorse Publishing

Skyhorse Publishing books may be purchased in bulk at special discounts for sales promotion, corporate gifts, fund-raising, or educational purposes. Special editions can also be created to specifications. For details, contact the Special Sales Department, Skyhorse Publishing, 307 West 36th Street, 11th Floor, New York, NY 10018 or info@skyhorsepublishing.com.

Skyhorse® and Skyhorse Publishing® are registered trademarks of Skyhorse Publishing, Inc.®, a Delaware corporation.

Visit our website at www.skyhorsepublishing.com.

10 9 8 7 6 5 4 3 2

Library of Congress Cataloging-in-Publication Data is available on file.

Cover design by Rain Saukas

Print ISBN: 978-1-63450-560-4
Ebook ISBN: 978-1-5107-0158-8

Printed in China

Dedication

This book is dedicated to all the hard working parents who sacrifice their time, energy, and resources to raise the future of our country.

It doesn't take a village to raise a child—it takes a parent.

"The most important thing that parents can teach their children is how to get along without them."

— Frank Clark

Table of Contents

Table of Contents

Introduction

"Tell me and I forget, teach me and I may remember, involve me and I learn."

—Benjamin Franklin

Deciding what projects to include in this book was one of the hardest things I have done as an author. Not knowing the age or temperament of future readers preclude some very neat projects, however, I do believe that learning how to control things that are potentially dangerous (such as fire and power tools) is a vital component of growing up.

I did enlist the help of my wife (who is a middle school special education teacher), my mom (who is a nationally board certified middle school teacher), as well as my limited experience teaching after school programs in order to select projects that would interest middle school-aged children—as well as to include some that would challenge older elementary-aged children with good adult supervision. Some projects may even interest a bored teenager.

You may notice that there are more kitchen-related projects than I normally include in a project book. This is done purposely, as it seems to me that cooking is a great way to introduce the concepts of self-confidence, independence, and attention to detail. I only began to gain confidence as a DIYer when I learned to make such "scary" items as cheese, linked sausages, and flavored vinegars. I would hope that this process can be started by completing fun campfire desserts like roasted Rolo marshmallows.

My wife uses cooking in her classroom because she believes that cooking helps introduce math and science concepts such as measurements and cause/effect.

If I could redo any of the mistakes of my childhood or early adulthood I would take a greater interest in working with my elders. My grandfather was a mechanical genius. He could create functional objects in any medium; he could weld, plumb, build, run heavy equipment, as well as use precision machine tools. He could repair almost anything—and when I could have learned at the knee of a master tradesman I preferred to sit in the air conditioned house and watch cable.

I am not an expert in child raising, but I know that kids need skills, they need to gain confidence by doing. And as a I have a duty to get my son out of the house and into a mess of dirt, grease, and wood shavings so that he had a chance to learn what he can do if he sets his mind to a task.

In the end, this book is very similar in nature to my other project books. There is an open secret that I believe that the actual projects are not nearly as important as the process that occurs when you actually work them with your children.

Please work these projects *with* your children, not *for* your children. It does not matter if the end result is not pretty, or even if it works. What this book is about is allowing kids the opportunity to expand their abilities and grow their self-confidence.

Introduction

No matter what your parenting style, skills, or philosophy, it is my belief that as parents we owe it to both our children and the world as a whole to ensure our fledglings learn the following skills (at a minimum) before they leave the nest:

- How to take responsibly for their actions
- How to work both singly and as a member of a team
- How to learn
- How to both take and give orders
- How to think for themselves and question authority
- How to manage their time to get necessary tasks accomplished by the deadlines
- How to tell the difference between a want and a need
- How to use basic tools for repairs
- How to cook more than microwaveable meals and ramen—to include shopping and meal planning
- How to clean
- How to be frugal
- How to budget and manage money—to include staying out of debt

It is my hope that the projects in this book help you teach these things to your children in a fun and accessible way.

How to Use This Book

Not knowing the age, skill level, or preferences of your child, I cannot recommend starting at chapter one and working through this book sequentially as I normally suggest.

If you have already incubated a love of cooking in your child you may want to start with the more interesting cooking projects, or avoid them until you and your children complete more mechanical projects.

Or you just may take a hands-off approach and give your kid the book and see what *they* want to try first. That's how my mom raised me; she gave me lots of cool project books and then stood back and helped me as needed.

No matter what order you decide to work this book, what is important is that you do the projects with your child. Let them explore, make decisions, and use tools. Guide them, help them, but both of you will enjoy and gain more from these projects if you let your kids experiment—even if they "fail."

PROJECT 1

BOTTLE CAP CANDLE

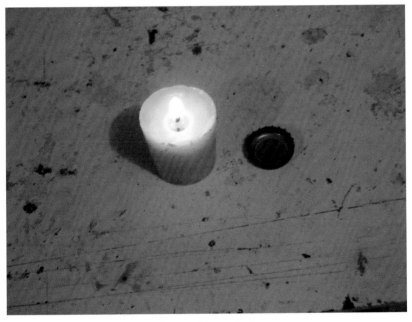

The Materials

Simple beeswax candles are very easy to make, last a long time, don't smoke or leave soot, and make a very clear light.

However, they can be large and take up too much space to put in small survival or bug out kits.

Our first project in this book is to recycle household scrap into a very small candle that fits very well in minimalist survival kits in addition to weighing next to nothing.

I find that it is very easy to construct these from the wax drippings from a burning candle, but you can make them in bulk by microwaving a small amount of wax in a Pyrex container (the wax will be extremely hot so do not use plastic).

This is definitely a project that requires adult supervision—but it is a guaranteed hit with pre-teens. I have never known an eleven- or twelve-year-old that did not like playing with fire . . .

Material:

- Wicking material—about ½ inch of cotton or other natural fiber string per candle
- Metal bottle cap
- Wax. I use beeswax, because it is easily available to me, but paraffin wax can also be used and can be purchased at almost any grocery store near the canning supplies.

Procedure:

1. Put your cap upside down on your working surface.
2. Place a drop of hot wax in the center of the cap.
3. Place one end of your string into the wax to set it in place.
4. Fill the cap up with wax.
5. Let cool, and put in your emergency kit with a lighter or other simple fire starter.

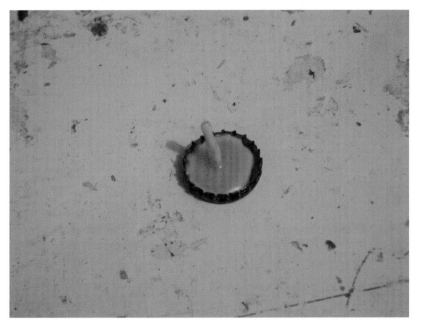

Finished Candle

Lessons Learned:

This project shows how to reduce, reuse, and recycle to make something that could be quite useful in a disaster.

PROJECT 2

BOTTLE CAP FISHING LURE

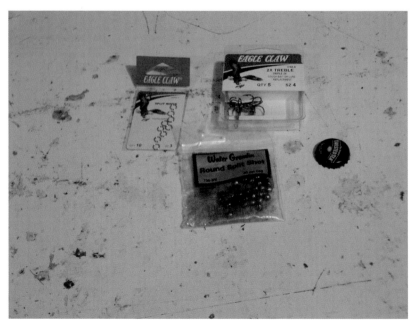

The Materials

Growing up, I used to like to go fishing. I was very bad at it, and since I always lost expensive fishing lures faster than I could earn enough money to replace them, my Dad rarely took me.

One day while scrolling through online videos in search of the end of the Internet, I found a really neat method of making fishing lures out of metal bottle tops. I was amazed at how neat the idea was, and immediately set about to make one for myself.

This is an easy project for a teenager or a skillful preteen. If strength is an issue with bending the bottle cap, the careful use of pliers can help. As I went about making this project the hardest part was drilling the holes. If needed, using a vice or a hammer to flatten the ends of the cap makes it much easier to drill, but be careful not to smash it too much or the split shot won't rattle inside the cap.

Materials:
- Beer/soda bottle top
- Split rings
- BBs or small split shot
- Treble hook
- Tools are simple also:
  - o Hammer and small nail/Drill and small bit
  - o Pliers

Procedure:
- Using your fingers, press the sides of the cap until it buckles.
- Before pushing the two ends together, place a couple BBs or shot into the cavity, so that they can rattle.

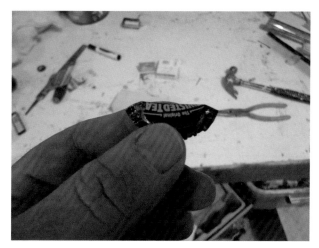

Smash Cap in half and drill hole in one end

1. Carefully drill or punch a hole at either end of the folded cap. It may help to slightly flatten the ends with your pliers.
2. Thread a split ring into each hole.
3. Thread a Treble hook into one of the split rings.
4. Go fishing.

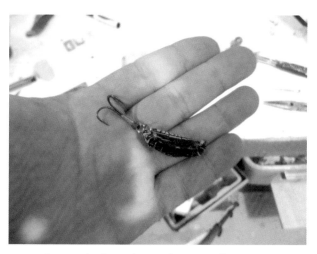

Attach hook using split ring

Lessons Learned:

This project builds on the previous project, by showing how a flexible mind can see new uses for items that may be outside of their designated use.

It also helps develop the skills to recognize new uses for common materials—which is vital to growing a flexible mind.

It also shows how resourcefulness can save money—which can be reinforced with a trip to the sporting goods store and showing how much money was saved by building a lure rather than buying one.

Bonus Tip

I have a hard time keeping things organized in my tackle box. It is almost as big a problem as the lost lures I get stuck in logs, weeds, and tree branches.

I have found that by using small safety pins, I can keep my fish hooks together by size in my fishing tackle. This trick also helps me to avoid getting stuck as I try to get lures and other tackle out of the box.

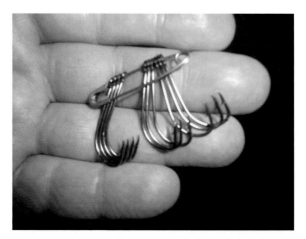

Keep hooks together using safety pins

PROJECT 3

DEHYDRATED TOOTHPASTE DOTS

Here is a quick tip for backpacking or camping where space and weight is a premium. I also find that my son thinks they are mints, so he chews them whenever his momma lets him have some.

This is a very easy project that someone as young as kindergarten age can accomplish. My toddler has helped me with this project, but he got more toothpaste on the wall than he did as nice neat dots on the parchment.

He also thinks the dots are candy, so that was another consideration . . . .

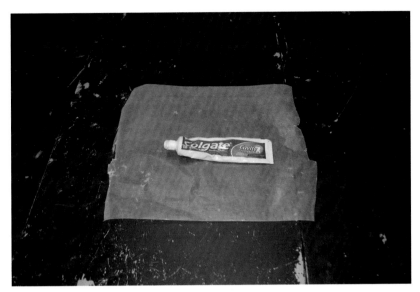

Simple Ingredients

Material:

- Paste Toothpaste (non-fluoride if you plan on swallowing the dots when done)
- Parchment paper
- Dehydrator (or oven with a cookie sheet if you do not have a dehydrator)
- Baking soda
- Small Ziploc bag

Procedure:

1. To make a chewable, single use, dry toothpaste "mint," lay out parchment and make rows of toothpaste spots.

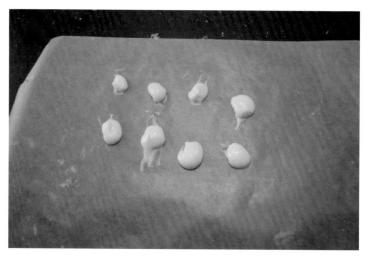

Make toothpaste balls

2. Allow to dry for 2–4 days.
3. Sprinkle baking soda on top to keep from sticking.
4. Repackage in small bags.

To use:

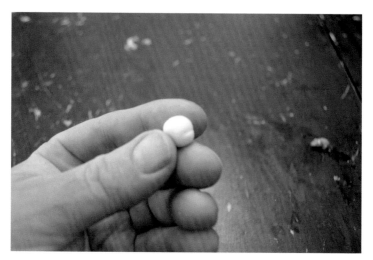

Pop dried ball into your mouth

Pop one dot in your mouth, chew, then add a small amount of water in your mouth and start brushing.

Lessons Learned:

Besides the obvious benefit of reinforcing personal hygiene, it introduces the process of dehydration, as well as allowing a conversation about the benefits of thinking ahead.

The time it takes to complete this project saves time and effort during later camping trips.

Note:

This is not a long term storage project—these dots should be used within a few weeks.

PROJECT 4

KEYCHAIN
FERROCERIUM ROD

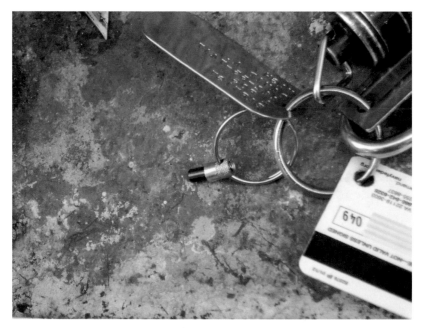

Finished project

If you are a welder, plumber, or just familiar with torches, you are probably familiar with the friction sparkers used to light propane or acetylene torches. I have found that they are also useful as emergency fire source that you can add to your keychain.

What make the sparkers work are small ferrocerium rods that are held in a small threaded brass fitting. These rods are replaceable, and normally when you buy a sparker you get five or six of them in the package for around five dollars.

It is quite easy to drill through the brass fitting, and if you use a small drill bit and a vise you can quickly drill a small hole through the end of the sparker.

If you thread this on a keychain you will always have the means to start a fire. It weighs fractions of an ounce—only a couple of grains (4,000 grains to a pound) and is tiny enough not to get in the way.

This is a great project for a mini survival kit, and I have one of these on my keychain. It takes virtually no space and adds an unnoticeable amount of weight but it does make me feel a little more comfortable with my survival ability.

My father was a State Park Ranger, so I grew up in the woods. This fuelled my obsession with building survival kits. I can't help but imagine there are a lot of ten- to fourteen-year-olds out there that would love to build a survival kit and use the tools in it to start a campfire.

Material:
- Ferrocerium striker for welding torches
- Split ring
- Knife

- Tinder (Tinder is easily combustible material that will glow under a shower of sparks. I like to use a very fine steel wool or cotton balls pulled apart)

Tools:
- Vise
- Drill
- ⅛-inch or smaller drill bit (depending on the size of your key ring)

Procedure:
1. Place sticker tip in vise to securely hold it while drilling.
2. Using the ⅛-inch drill bit, drill through brass base, taking care not to drill into the base of the ferrocium rod itself, or break through the base of the striker.
3. Thread the striker onto your keychain.

To use:
1. Find tinder (0000-grade steel wool works great) and fluff it until it makes a loose bed to catch sparks.
2. Bring striker down closely to the tinder so that any sparks will land in the center of your combustible tender.
3. Using a knife, bear down on the striker and slide the blade down (in a scraping not cutting action).
4. Once the tinder catches a spark and begins to glow, gently blow it until it can be used to ignite a fire, much as a match would be used.

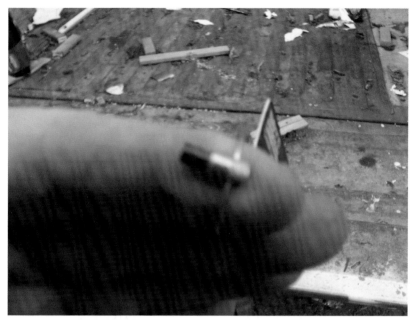

Small brass-tipped welding igniter tip

Lessons Learned:

Gaining the ability to make fire, and the trust implied with gaining this ability, is a rite of passage that is being lost in the modern world. There is something primal that is triggered by a campfire. It also calls for a frank discussion about responsibility, and that having the ability to do something does not always mean that something should be done. It calls for an understanding of cause and effect, and how careless handling of such a powerful tool as fire can cause irreversible damage.

Plus someone gets to use power tools . . .

Note:

Proper, safe, and conscious use of power tools is needed to complete this project. It may be appropriate for the adult to drill the hole, and the child to place it on the split ring.

This is also a difficult way to start fire; it takes practice and a concerted effort to strike a spark and catch it in the tinder—which in itself is another lesson.

PROJECT 5

APPLE PANCAKES

One of the first things I learned to cook was a simple pancake. It was also the first thing I cooked with my son. I have great memories of a sticky-fingered, syrup-covered two-year-old learning to flip pancakes hand over hand with me.

Our first cooking project is a little more complex than simple pancakes, but I think it is easier. I also feel that the results are more dramatic to create something a little more dramatic and "cooler" than simple pancakes.

As an added benefit, this recipe is easily used with children of different skill levels. Young children can dump in premeasured ingredients and stir them in the bowl, while older children can easily make these delicious apple pancakes themselves.

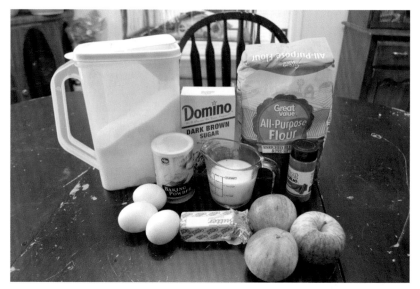

The Ingredients

Ingredients:

- 2 tablespoons butter
- 3 apples (peeled, cored and sliced into wedges)
- ¼ cup brown sugar
- ½ teaspoon cinnamon
- 3 large eggs
- ½ cup whole milk (reduced fat or almond milk may be substituted)
- 2 tablespoons flour
- ¼ teaspoon baking powder
- powdered sugar, for dusting (optional)

Tools:

- Measuring cups
- 2 mixing bowls
- Knife/apple corer

- Spoon
- 12- or 13-inch cast iron skillet or other oven safe pan

Procedure:

1. Preheat oven to 375 degrees.

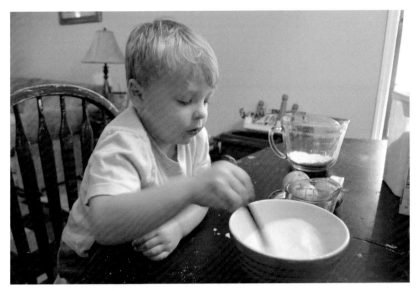

Mix the dry ingredients first

2. In a medium mixing bowl, mix the flour and baking powder.
3. In a separate bowl, whisk together 3 eggs and ½ cup milk.
4. Add egg/milk mixture into bowl with dry ingredients and stir until you get a batter (a few lumps is fine).
5. Combine brown sugar and cinnamon but do not add to batter.
6. In a skillet, melt the butter on medium heat.

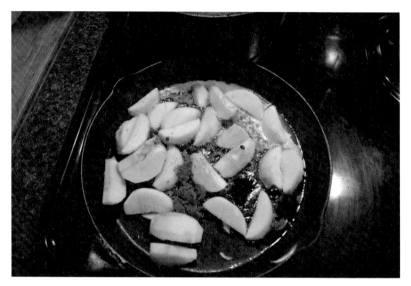

Cook the apples with sugar until soft

7. Add the apple slices and 1 tablespoon of the brown sugar mixture to the hot skillet and cook until soft, stirring as necessary. This should take about 5 minutes.

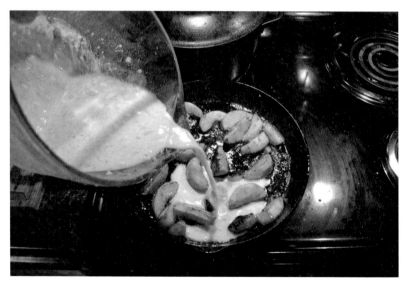

Carefully pour in batter without moving apples

8. Turn off the stove top, and gently and slowly pour the batter over the apples so as to keep the apples evenly distributed in the pan.
9. Sprinkle the remaining brown sugar on top of the batter.
10. Bake at 375 until the pancake mix puffs up, which should take 18–20 minutes.
11. If desired, dust the finished pancake with a little powdered sugar.

Yield:

Serves 2–3

Lessons Learned:

Cooking teaches cause and effect, following directions, the use of measurement, and delayed gratification. Easy projects like this introduce the concepts, while building self-confidence and pride of accomplishment.

PROJECT 6

DUCT TAPE TIP

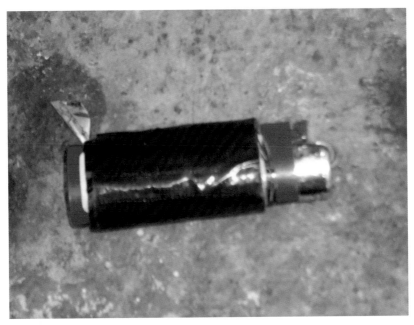

A water bottle works well, but you can use almost anything you keep in your pocket.

This project is another (the key chain lighter was the first) "everyday carry" item.

It has long been a common trick among backpackers to wrap some duct tape around their water bottle or lighter so that they always have a couple feet readily available for quick repairs.

I find that having some duct tape with me in the things that I carry everyday helps me stay prepared. When hiking, I can use it on "hotspots" to prevent blisters, and it's invaluable for survival when making things like plastic water stills and bags. However, since I spend most of my time in an office, I tend to use my duct tape in more normal ways.

Once I got used to always having some duct tape with me, I took the concept one step further so that I would always have some duct tape with me even if I only had my keys.

Material:
- Old ink pen or ⅛ inch diameter plastic pipe about 4 inches long
- Duct Tape
- String—I used a paracord monkey fist
- Split ring keychain

Tools:
- Saw or small pipe cutter
- Knife

Procedure:
1. Start by taking an old ink pen that is no longer serviceable and cut the ends off with a pipe cutter, leaving a hollow tube as long as the roll of tape was wide. Alternatively you can use a small diameter pipe.

2. Wrap about 4 feet of tape around the tube—in essence creating a mini-roll of black duct tape.
3. Thread the string through the pipe tying a knot on one end and the other to a keychain split ring. I used a monkey fist that I keep on my keychain.

Now you have a captive roll of tape that is always with you. It takes no extra space, and adds very little weight.

Lessons Learned:

This is a simple little project, and while it only takes a minute to do, it starts the process of thinking about what simple steps can a person take NOW that will make life easier LATER.

The first time a problem arises that your child solves with their stash of tape opens the door to a conversation about the benefits of saving for the future and being prepared.

PROJECT 7

IMPROVISED KNIFE SHARPENING TIP

Today I offer you an improvised knife-sharpening tip. Improvised means it is not as good as a normal method of using a whetstone or other sharpener, but that it will work in a pinch.

If you take a ceramic coffee mug or bowl and flip it upside down you will notice a ring where there is no glaze.

It is possible to use this ring to sharpen your knife blade just as you would use a ceramic sharpening rod.

I have tried this, and it does leave residue on the ceramic ring, and it does sharpen the blade.

I would stay away from using this on my high quality knives, but it's perfect for when you are out camping and you need to sharpen a knife right then. It's a good idea to keep in the back of your mind.

Hopefully this can help you in the future.

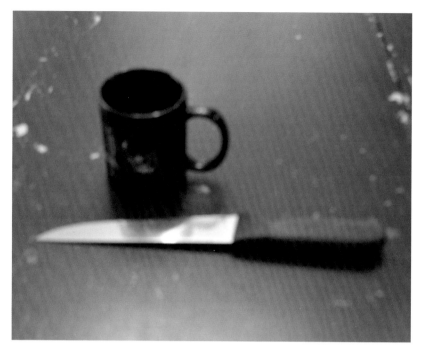

The Materials

Material:
- Knife

Tools:
- Ceramic coffee mug

Procedure:
1. Flip a ceramic coffee cup over and find the unglazed ring that is left from the firing process.
2. Use this ring like a whetstone, by sliding the knife blade along the unglazed ring as if you were slicing it.

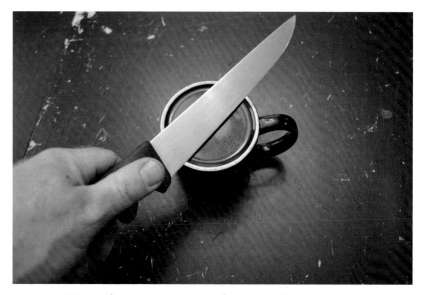

Use the cup as a sharpening stone

3. Go slowly and gently, matching the angle of the knife blade to the angle of grind on the blade so you only remove metal from the cutting edge and not the side of the knife blade.

Lessons Learned:

This project teaches that once you understand how something works, you can apply that knowledge in new ways. Ceramic knife sharpeners work by removing small amounts of metal from a blade, and the unglazed ring on the bottom of a ceramic mug can do the same thing.

This project also teaches that improvised is not always better.

An improvised knife sharpener will never be as easy, as fast, or do as good a job as a specially designed piece of equipment, but becoming adaptable and resilient means knowing how to make do and being able to determine when it is best NOT to improvise.

Note:

This project involves using sharp knives, it is vital that care is taken to ensure that the knife is sharpened AWAY from the body, and that the fingers holding the mug are kept well away from the blade.

This project is only suitable for children with a high level of maturity and adult supervision.

PROJECT 8

PARACORD CARABINER SPOOL

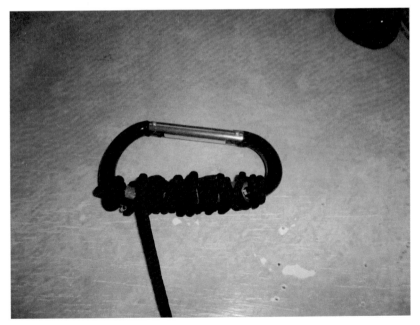

The finished spool

This is a really easy project that is very useful for outdoorsmen of all types. It is just a way of carrying cordage in a way that is easily accessible.

If you can get a section of PVC pipe around a carabiner and spool 550 or tethering cord around it, you can use the carabiner to attach to the outside of your pack when not needed, and either spool from your pack, or detach it and use from the spool. Heck, you could even hold the free end, and use the carabiner spool as a weight to throw over a tree for things like hanging bear bags.

The D shaped carabiners will have the most room for carrying Paracord. The diameter of the carabiner tubing should be slightly smaller than the interior spool diameter to reduce wobble and to give you more room for spooled cord.

Material:
- Large "D" ring carabiner
- ½-inch PVC pipe
- Cord

Tools:
- Saw
- Sandpaper
- Tape

Procedure:
1. Cut a 3" section of ½" PVC pipe to use as a spool.
2. This won't fit directly on the carabiner; you need to cut a slit down the center of the pipe. (Do not cut the pipe into two halves; only cut down one side so you can pry it open.)

3. Force the cut apart so you can slide it over the carabiner body. Ensure you use the non-opening end.
4. Ensure the pipe can spin freely around the carabiner.
5. Next, wrap as much paracord on the spool as you can, (probably about 40 feet worth), you should stop while you are still be able to open the carabiner gate just enough to slip it over nylon webbing/PALS/MOLLE attachment point on your bag, backpack, strap, or vest.

Lessons Learned:

This project reinforces the concept of mental flexibility and the benefits of looking at the function of materials outside of their designated use.

Note:

The use of a saw to split the PVC tubing necessitates adult supervision.

PROJECT 9

CAMPFIRE POPCORN

My household buys popcorn in twenty-five or fifty gallon bulk bags at the local warehouse store rather than in individual microwavable bags. We do this because it is so much cheaper to buy in bulk, but also because, if necessary, popcorn can be ground into some resemblance of cornmeal.

It is likely that you can buy a bulk bag of popcorn for what a box of two of microwavable popcorn costs.

The issue is one of convenience—not quality. It is my experience that freshly popped corn made over a stove or campfire is much better than popcorn made in a microwave.

Since we have a project or two that revolves around fire-starting, I believe that this book should share projects to make that fire useful—otherwise a child can lose sight that fire is a tool to be controlled and used appropriately.

Popping corn over a campfire is a really cool way of using fire to cook food—and it is pretty tasty as well.

Ingredients:

- 1 Teaspoon Popcorn
- 1 Teaspoon Oil
- Butter
- Salt

Tools:

- Heavy Duty foil
- Fire
- Stick
- Cotton String

Procedure:

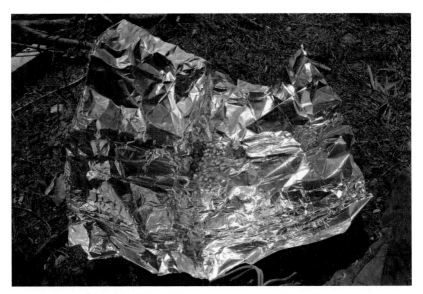

Put oil and popcorn in center of a square of foil

1. In the center of an 18" x 18" square of heavy-duty or doubled foil, place one teaspoon of oil and one teaspoon of popcorn.
2. Bring foil corners together to make a pouch.
3. Seal the edges by folding, but allow room for the popcorn to pop.

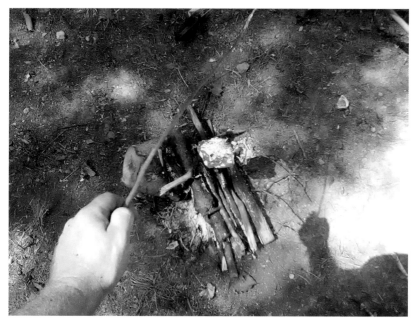

Hold over coals

4. Tie each pouch to a long stick with a string and hold the pouch over the hot coals.
5. Shake constantly until all the corn has popped. Season with butter and salt.

Campfire Popcorn

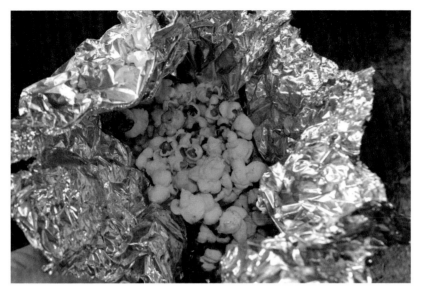

Popcorn in foil

Yield:

Serves one

Lessons Learned:

Cooking over a campfire reinforces that fire is a tool, and that with knowledge and skill dangerous things can be safely controlled and made useful.

Comparing the costs of home cooked popcorn with the per unit cost of microwavable popcorn introduces the cost of convenience

The superior taste and pride of accomplishment that comes with cooking teaches the contrast between effort and convenience, furthering the development of self-discipline.

PROJECT 10

CAMPFIRE ROLO MARSHMALLOWS

This project is also one to be done over a campfire.

Instead of roasting plain marshmallows over a campfire, poke a hole in the center of the marshmallow and insert a mini Rolo.

(If desired, you could substitute plain chocolate or other mini candy bar).

The caramel and chocolate will melt inside the marshmallow and fundamentally transform the treat.

The end result is similar to a s'more with caramel.

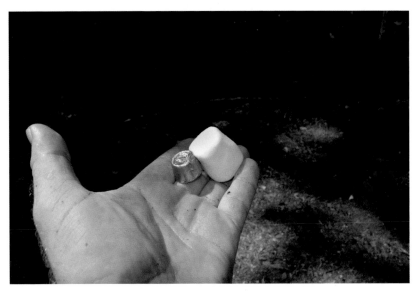

The Ingredients

Ingredients:
- 1 bag of large marshmallows
- 1 bag of mini Rolo candy (or other candy bar—I like mini Snickers.)

Tools:
- Stick
- Fire

Procedure:
1. Poke a hole into the center of a marshmallow.

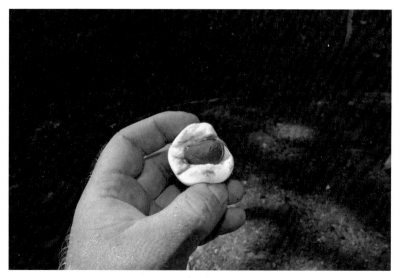

Stuff Rolo candy into marshmallow

2. Cram a small Rolo candy into the hole.
3. Push the marshmallow/Rolo onto the stick and roast over a fire.

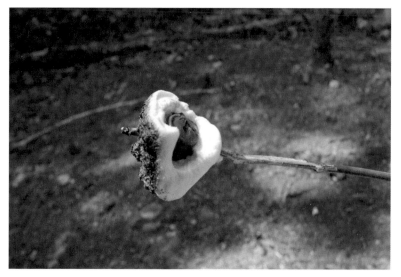

Char as desired

Yield:

Happy children

Lessons Learned:

Cooking over a campfire reinforces that fire is a tool, and that with knowledge and skill dangerous things can be safely controlled and made useful.

Using alternate candies also rewards imagination.

I know this is a not quite a full project, but it does support the real goal of the book, which is spending quality time with children while teaching them how to think.

I don't know of any better way to teach children creativity other than letting them see firsthand the benefit of trying new things. If your kids are in scouts or other youth orientated outdoor groups, I imagine they will show their friends this project at their very next outing. This will reinforce the benefit of knowing (and sharing) new things.

PROJECT 11

MOUNTAIN DEW APPLE DUMPLINGS

This is another dessert recipe that is easy enough for a middle school child to accomplish with a minimum of supervision, but tastes good enough that even an older child will be proud of the result.

I am forty(ish) and still have a feeling of pride when I share this recipe at potluck meals.

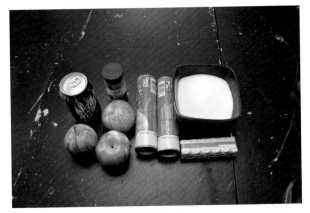

The Ingredients

Ingredients

- 2 cans crescent rolls
- 3–4 tart apples
- 1 ½ cups sugar
- ½ cup butter
- 1 teaspoon cinnamon
- 1 12-ounce can Mountain Dew soda (or generic)

Procedure

1. Grease, oil or spray a 9" x 13" baking dish or pan.
2. Preheat oven to 350 degrees F.
3. Peel and slice apples. I use one of those round cutters that core and slice in one shot. You will need at least one slice per crescent roll (I sometimes use two apple slices if they are particularly small).

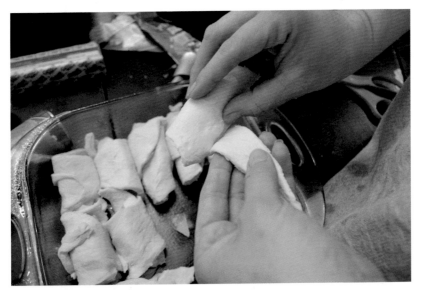

Wrap apple slices with crescent roll triangles

4. Roll each apple slice in a section of crescent roll.
5. Place rolled slices in pan, and put extras alongside. You want them all to fit nicely together without cramming them together, but still close enough for them to rise into one tasty mass.

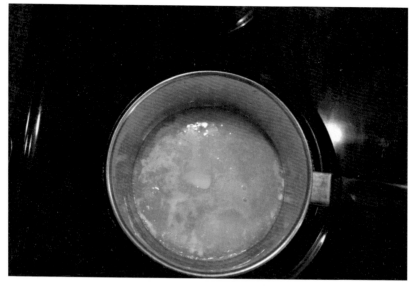

Melt butter, sugar, and cinnamon until the sugar is liquefied

6. Melt butter, add sugar and cinnamon, stir until the sugar is liquefied, and pour over apples.
7. Pour can of Mountain Dew over all.
8. Bake at 350 degrees for 45 minutes.

Enjoy with vanilla ice cream—tastes just like apple pie.

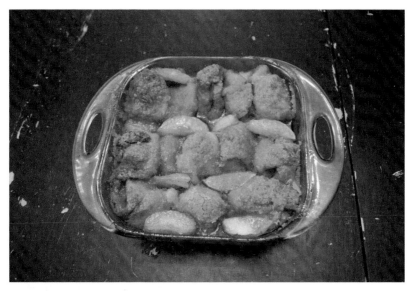

Finished dessert

Lessons Learned:

As a simple recipe with a sophisticated end result, this recipe teaches children the benefit of skill acquisition.

A little effort in the kitchen, combined with practice and a small amount of knowledge, gives a result that garners praise and allows a sense of worthy pride.

PROJECT 12

TUNA CAN CAKE

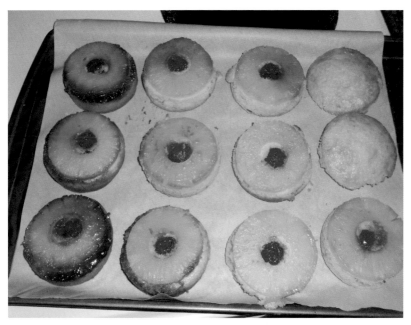

Individual Pineapple upside-down cakes

I like pineapple upside-down cake, but I don't make it often. We never end up eating the whole cake and I hate to see it wasted.

I first tried this recipe as an experiment in using cleaned out tuna cans (it grew out of the stove experiment in an earlier project book).

The result was much better than expected, and the individual portions were a hit, and allowed excess to be frozen for later use.

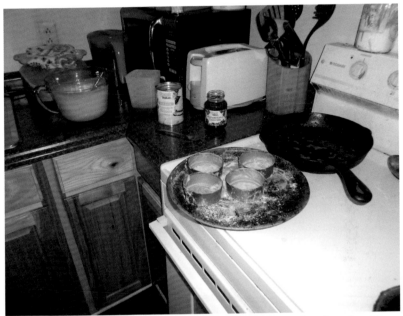

Greased and floured tuna cans ready for batter

Ingredients:

- Cake mix
- Egg*
- Oil*
- Flour*
- 1 can of Pineapple rings
- 1 jar cherries

*These ingredient amounts will depend upon the cake mix you purchase. Refer to the amounts listed on the box.

Tools:

- 6–12 cleaned tuna cans (the more you have the easier the project—I have done it with 4)
- Parchment paper
- Cookie sheet
- Mixing bowl
- Spoon
- Measuring cups
- Toothpick

Procedure:

1. Following the recipe on the cake mix box, mix the cake batter.
2. Preheat your oven as listed on the recipe.
3. A pineapple ring fits very well in a tuna can; place one ring into each tuna can.
4. Place a cherry in the center of each ring.
5. Fill each can ¾ full of the batter.
6. Place the filled tuna cans on a cookie sheet and bake for 15–20 minutes, or until a toothpick inserted into the cake comes out clean. (Time depends on many factors so check your cakes—I find that earlier batches cook faster as the oven cools from repeated openings.)
7. Dump the can over on a parchment paper-covered cookie sheet and refill until you have made enough individual cakes.
8. Let cool and enjoy.

Yield:

One can is a single serving

Lessons Learned:

This project is one of the most difficult recipes in this book, but the results are some of the best.

This teaches that reward requires effort, and that to achieve good results time must be spent mastering simple skills before attempting the more complex.

PROJECT 13

HARDTACK CRACKERS

Hardtack is basically a large hard cracker that was a staple of the civil war soldier's diet, however, while it was best known for its role in that conflict, hardtack had been used long before that war, and for feeding other groups such as sailors and outdoorsmen.

Hardtack has been used in various forms and using various grains as a base since the time of the Egyptian pharaohs, and it is still made today by a factory in Virginia for use in Alaska. Anyone who needs a shelf-stable, long-lasting, lightweight food should consider hardtack.

The secret to its success is that it has no fat to go rancid, and no moisture to cause it to spoil. The only ingredients are flour, salt, and water to form the dough. It is then rolled into ⅛ to ½ inch sheets and baked until the moisture is driven out.

The problem with hardtack is that it is hard. This hardness helps it travel well, but makes it hard to eat. Normally hardtack is crumbled into a soup or coffee and eaten as a mush, or it is soaked in brine and cooked, or cooked with meats in a skillet. Very seldom is it actually eaten as a whole unbroken cracker. This probably is why it was "affectionately" named teeth-breakers by some soldiers.

It's simple to make, and as a side note, it's the base of most dog biscuits . . . .

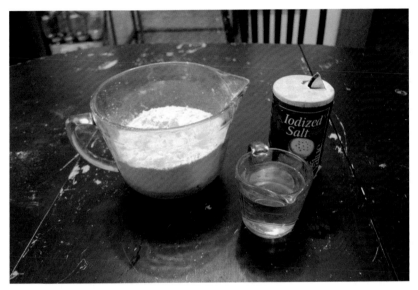

The Ingredients

Ingredients
- 6 cups flour
- 1 cup water
- 1 tablespoon salt

Tools:
- Rolling pin
- Fork
- Cookie sheet

- Mixing bowl
- Spoon
- Knife (a pizza cutter works well)

Procedure

1. Mix ingredients into a bowl and mix until a dough is formed.
2. Turn dough onto a floured surface.
3. Knead dough until thoroughly mixed.

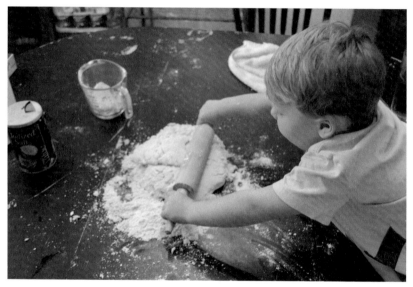

Roll out the dough

4. Roll out on a floured surface until about ⅛ inch thick (or thicker if desired).

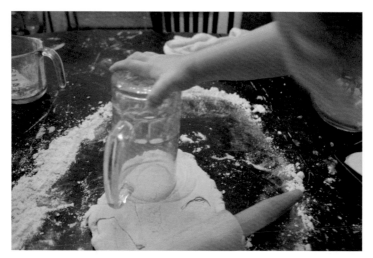

Cut out biscuits

5. Cut into biscuits—traditionally it was square, but I like mine round.

6. Use a fork to poke holes in the hardtack; this is not for looks, but to allow steam to escape while cooking and to ensure complete cooking.

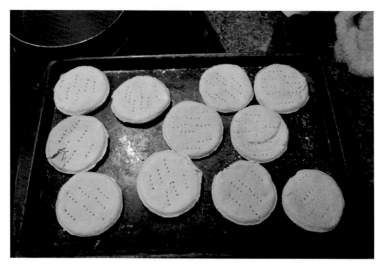

Bake until hard

7. Bake at 325 for at least an hour, turning over the hard tack once. Check to see that it is cooked through completely.
8. Remove from oven and let cool uncovered overnight to harden.
9. Traditionally, hardtack for naval use was traditionally baked another 3 times to ensure there was no moisture left.

Yield:

Several crackers that are the basis of a three-day subsistence ration for a single person.

Lessons Learned:

Hardtack is one recipe that I find all DIY preppers attempt at some point. By learning how to make this, I find that it teaches that all advancement is built from those that came before us, and that to become knowledgeable we must respect and understand the efforts of those that came before us and developed the techniques we may have come to take for granted.

PROJECT 14

TIN CAN GRILL

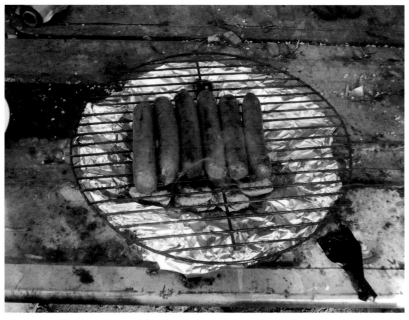

Tin can grill

Today's project is a small homemade grill made from a can, some foil, and a round charcoal grate.

This project works best with a #10 can, but like most of my projects, once you have the concept you can feel free to experiment based upon your needs and materials at hand.

This isn't the most efficient grill, but you can't beat the price, and once you're done with it, most everything is recyclable so all you have to keep is the round grate. This makes storage simple.

Materials:

- #10 can
- Aluminum foil
- Grate

Procedure:

1. Mark the top of the can into 10 equally wide segments.
2. Using tin snips cut along these marks until you have 10 strips that are ⅔ as long as the depth of the can (this leaves the bottom ⅓ in one piece to keep the round shape.
3. Bend these strips out so they radiate outwards. Do not press them all the way down; they should form a dish.
4. Place aluminum foil over the can, so that it forms a bowl supported by the 10 strips.
5. Insert charcoal into bowl, and light—take care not to use so much that the mound of fuel rises above the top of the bowl.
6. Place grate on grill, so that the metal strips support it.
7. Grill food and enjoy.

Lessons Learned:

This project reinforces the earlier skill of solving problems by looking at function and form to find materials that can be used outside of their design to create items that are needed.

It also reinforces the benefit of reusing and recycling rather than buying new.

PROJECT 15

PENNY BATTERY

This isn't a practical project, but it is a practical bit of knowledge to keep in the back of your head.

What we are making today is voltaic piles out of pennies, zinc coated washers, and bits of paper.

Each cell consisting of a penny, a washer, and a small square of wet paper produces up to about 0.8 volts, and you can stack multiple cells to create higher voltages.

I have done this with after-school groups with kids in kindergarten to fifth grade (with various depth of explanation) and it is very useful to introduce chemistry and the fun of DIY.

Some people use 1982–present pennies that have the copper coating sanded off as the zinc, but since it is illegal to deface US currency, I use zinc washers (well . . . to be honest I use zinc washers because it is MUCH easier).

If you want to do anything slightly resembling useful, you will need at least five cells. It would take a pile about the size of your living room and five feet tall to actually run your home, so lighting up a LED or sounding a small piezo electric buzzer are about the limits of this tech.

I have found more than five cells starts to get unwieldy, and trying to use electric tape to hold it together has stymied the video for some time—maybe using a plastic coin roll, or a length of plastic pipe may make this project easier.

A cell like this will only work about six hours or so, but it does show the potential to use chemistry knowledge to do useful work.

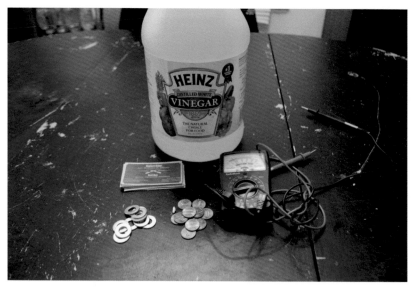

The Materials

Material:
- Pennies (or 1-inch copper strips cut into squares)
- Zinc washers
- Thin cardboard (I use old business cards)
- Vinegar

Tools:

- Wire
- Small light or buzzer
- Scissors to cut cardboard (optional)
- Tape (optional)
- Cup (optional)

Procedure:

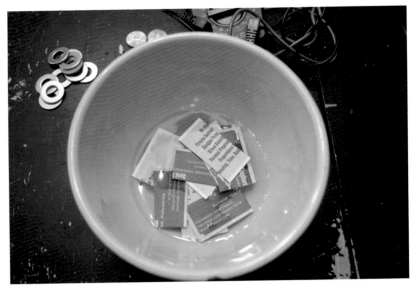

Cut cards into squares and soak in vinegar

1. Rip up a piece of thin cardboard (I use business cards, but something like a cereal box would probably work) into squares the approximately the size of a penny but slightly larger.
2. Soak the squares in vinegar or lemon juice.

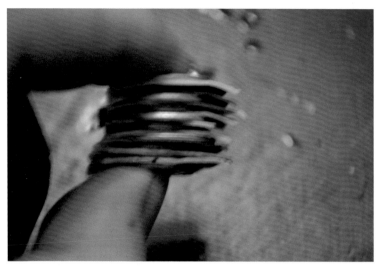

Layer Penny, Paper, Zinc

3. Layer in the following sequence:
   3.1. Penny
   3.2. Soaked Paper
   3.3. Zinc

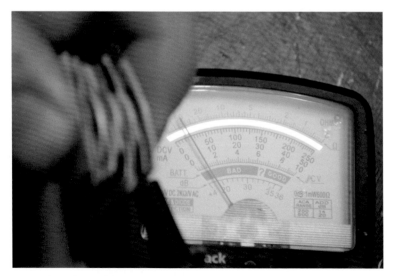

Multiple cells will make a volt meter move

4. This makes one cell. To make useable voltage, stack more cells on top of each other until you can use the wires to light a small bulb or make a small buzzer sound.

Lessons Learned:

This project teaches that science is useful and can be fun. In my experience most kids like school until social convention teaches them that they should not like it.

I figured out early on that I learned better when I knew why I had to learn something. Trigonometry or chemistry was not fun if it was taught as things I needed to remember for a test, but were awesome when I realized that I could take that knowledge to DO things.

PROJECT 16

CORK KEYCHAIN

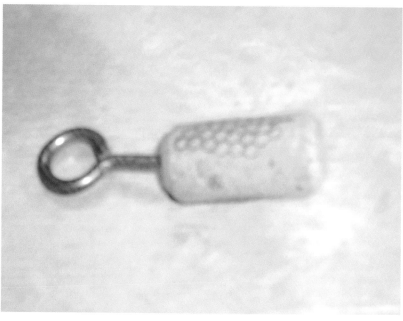

Finished Keychain

Having fun on the water is something most kids love to do. Boating, rafting, tubing, or just wading in a creek are all fun ways to spend hot summer days.

However, a good way to ruin the fun is to see your keys sink into the murky depths. Many people prevent this by purchasing a floating keychain for their boat and truck keys.

Fortunately, you don't have to purchase a floating fob, as you can easily make one with a cork and a small eyehook.

This won't hold a maintenance man's key ring above water, but it will hold your boat, truck, and house keys.

Material:
1. Cork
2. Small Eyehook
3. Key ring

Procedure:
1. Get a long shanked eyehook, and screw it through the center of the cork.
2. Attach a split ring to the eye.
3. Thread on your keys.

Lessons Learned:
Besides thinking ahead to prevent problems rather than having to deal with the consequences, this project makes a great gift for a boat owner.

PROJECT 17

MASON JAR BUTTER

For most of us, making your own butter is not really that efficient, but it is a neat project that introduces kids to the type of work that our forefathers used to do.

This project is one that I have done at several schools to introduce children to homesteading concepts.

I find that kids really enjoy making their own butter, and using a blender makes this project much easier than shaking the jar until butter is formed.

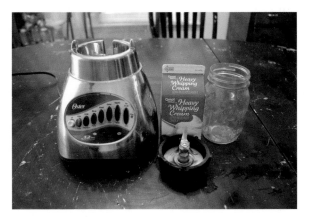

The Ingredients

Ingredients
- 1 pint heavy whipping cream, very cold
- Pinch of salt, optional

Tools:
- Mason Jar
- Blender
- Spoon
- Bowl
- Strainer

Procedure
1. Cool the jar by refrigerating the empty jar for at least 1 hour.
2. Fill the jar halfway with the cream.
3. Screw the blender top onto the top of the mason jar and pulse until butter forms. (Alternatively you can shake the jar violently for 15 to 20 minutes.)
4. Pour into a strainer set over a bowl. The chunks in the strainer are butter, and the liquid in the bowl is butter-milk.
5. Turn the butter into a clean bowl and cover with very cold water.

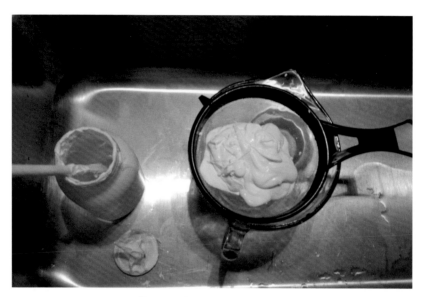

Pour into strainer

6. Pour into a strainer, discarding the liquid.
7. Continue rinsing the butter with very cold water until the water runs clear. (The cloudy water is buttermilk which will make the butter turn sour.)
8. When the water is clear, knead the butter using a wooden spoon to press out any remaining water or milk.
9. Discard this liquid.
10. If desired, add salt to the butter. (Salted butter will keep longer.)
11. Transfer the butter to a clean container for keeping, pressing with a wooden spoon or spatula to dispel any air bubbles. Refrigerate until ready to use.

Lessons Learned:

This experiment allows kids to see scientific magic unfold before their eyes. Heavy cream is what is called an "emulsion." An emulsion exists when tiny droplets of one type of liquid are floating around in another type of liquid that does not like to mix with the first. In the case of heavy cream, tiny globules of fat are suspended in mostly water. By blending the heavy cream, you are forcing the fat globules to slam into one another. If they hit each other with enough force, they will stick together, and the fat collection will become larger and large with each extra globule. After enough blending, the fat globules form a chunk of butter.

PROJECT 18

NEWSPAPER SEED POT

My experience says that simply buying a can of "emergency" seeds and planning on creating a garden in the event of a disaster is not a good plan. Gardening is a skill that only comes from doing it year after year.

While it is easiest to start your garden education using seedlings, at some point you will want to learn to grow plants from seed.

While you can buy all manner of seed starting tools and gadgets, I find that handmade newspaper seed pots are easiest and provide the best value.

I started making seed pots using a little wooden tool that cost about $20, but after a couple of years I realized that a glass bottle works just as well, and is a lot cheaper.

To create the paper pot you simply wrap a newspaper strip around the wooden dowel, then fold the bottom of the paper inward. Next you place the newspaper wrapped pot maker in the stand that's included with the kit and give it a little twist to seal the bottom of the pot.

Slide off, fill with soil, plant seed—entire pot is planted in garden so as not to disturb root ball.

That's it—pretty simple.

I did tend to cut too wide of a strip—easily remedied by ripping off excess in a similar fashion to how some of us menfolk try to wrap Christmas gifts and cut away the excess paper around the edges (that might just be me).

I also like to really grind the base into the wooden mandrel; I don't know if it made a better seal, but I felt like it did.

It felt a little awkward to pull the flimsy pot off of the wooded die, but once it was filled with dirt, I was very satisfied with the process. I think this is a great product, for what it is, and for what it would take to make one (for those of us without a wood lathe) is a good value and I wish I would have bought one several years ago.

Now all I have to hope for is that my seeds grow and I can harvest some vegetables this year because I don't know how much more I can spend on gardening tools, seeds, and raised beds without showing some harvest . . .

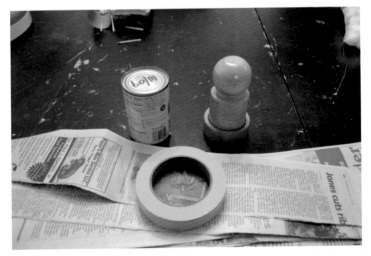

The Materials (can on left, commercial pot maker on right)

Material:

- Newspaper
- Masking tape (optional)

Tools:

- Scissors (or with practice you can rip newsprint by hand)
- Can, glass jar, or a thick glass bottle
- Hard surface to press against

Procedure:

1. Cut a strip of newspaper 4–6 inches wide—I normally rip a sheet of newspaper into 3 sections lengthwise.
2. Wrap the newspaper strips around the can or wooden mold, leaving enough overhanging the bottom of the can that is a little more than the radius of the bottle bottom.
3. Tape the edge if desired (I normally don't).

4. Fold the edges of the overhanging paper similar to folding up a paper coin roll.
5. Tape the bottom, if desired (again, I normally don't).
6. Firmly press the can bottom of glass bottle against a hard flat surface and rotate can to "smash" the roll shut.
7. Gently slide the rolls off and fill with dirt.

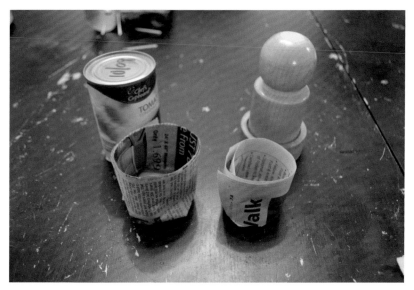

Completed pots

Lesson Learned:

Growing plants from seeds is a common school experiment and opens the door to discussions on biology and ecology, but I like using this to talk about all the things that have to happen to create the food we eat. It fosters a sense of connectedness and an understanding of how complicated (and how simple) things are.

PROJECT 19

RAIN BARREL

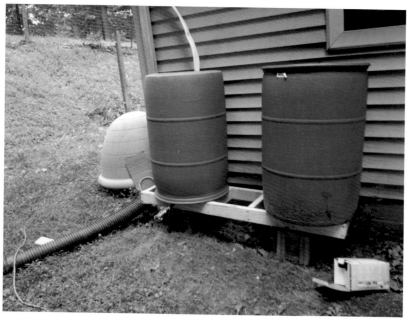

Finished rain barrel

Water is the second most important resource to sustaining human life. Without a steady supply of clean water, a person would die in a matter of days. For this reason I think it is important to be able to provide some measure of personal drinking water.

For ecological (and economical) reasons, I like to collect rain water—and while I don't normally drink this collected water, it does do a good job of watering my garden.

This project is one of the easiest ways to turn a 55-gallon plastic drum into a rain catchment system. It is much easier than climbing into the bottom of a drum to attach a faucet, and it works with closed top drums that are easier to find.

Materials:

- Surplus plastic 55-gallon drum that held coconut oil—use a food grade barrel. A new potable water barrel will cost several times more than a food grade surplus drum, and will not make the water "potable" since the roof, gutter, and other parts are not certified food grade.
- ½-inch long ¾-inch pipe nipple
- 90 degree elbow
- 6-inch long ¾ pipe nipple
- ¾ drain
- ¾-inch coupler
- Teflon tape
- Tools
- Drill with a ¾ bit

Procedure

1. Clean drum to remove any prior contents.
2. Use Teflon tape on all connections for a watertight seal.
3. Screw ½ nipple and 6-inch nipple into the 90 degree elbow.
4. Screw coupler on free end of the 6-inch pipe nipple.
5. Drill a ¾-inch hole in the center of the bung.

6. Screw ½ nipple into bung, tighten, but ensure that the pipe extends perpendicular to an imaginary centerline extending through the bung and along the radius of the barrel.

7. With the bung facing up, screw the drain into the coupler until it is tight and the open end of the couple is also facing up.

8. Take the drum outside, flip over and support with blocks or other stand so that the drain is facing down and the barrel is level.

9. Drill a hole as close in diameter to the water collection system hose as possible in the top of the barrel as it sits on site. Make sure the hose coming from your water collector will reach your hole. For aesthetic purposes I try to make this hole as close to the gutter as possible

10. Insert drain hose into hole.

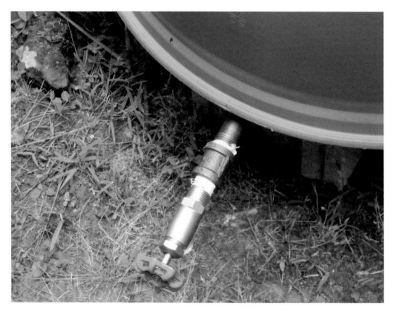

Finished valve

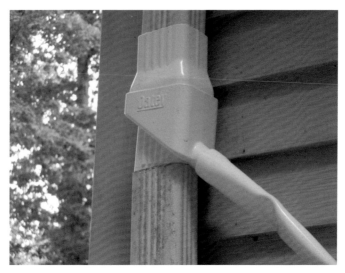

Diverter installed on gutter

If using a gutter diverter like the one I used, it will have instructions for how to cut your existing gutter system and install it. You do not have to use the model I did, as there are several on the market.

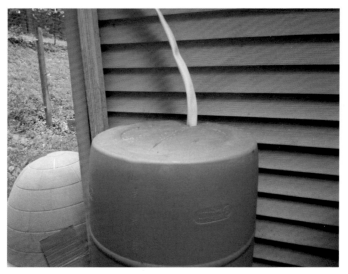

Hose from diverter into barrel

I try to keep the inlet hole as small as possible to keep mosquitos from being able to lay eggs in the water barrel. (If the water is for non-potable uses like watering gardens, you may want to add some mosquito fish to the barrel. If you do this you will be amazed at how few mosquitos you will have around the house after a few cycles of the tiny fish eating all the mosquito larva.)

Lesson Learned:

Any water discussion can lead to a discussion about the difference between a want and a need as well as what is (and is not) important in life.

This is also a good way to introduce the use of power tools, as the measurements are not critical, and there are only a few holes to be drilled.

PROJECT 20

TWO TYPES OF HOMEMADE FIRE STARTERS

The ability to make fire is an essential survival skill, and when looking at the history of the development of civilization, we could not have developed without mastering fire.

While fire making can be dangerous, it is that danger that must be addressed in order to create well-adjusted children that can handle the world's dangers resiliently.

In order to learn to master fire, we are going to make two different types of fire starters that act as "training wheels" to help create fire easily.

Type 1—Petroleum Jelly Soaked Cotton Ball

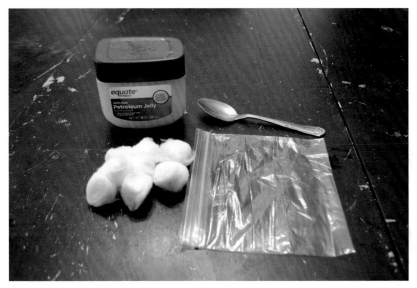

Type 1 Materials

This type of fire starter works very well, and the tiny filaments in the cotton balls work very well to collect sparks from things like the earlier Keychain Ferrocerium Rod.

Material:
- Cotton balls
- 100% Petroleum Jelly (non-mentholated)

Tools:
- Ziploc bag

Procedure:

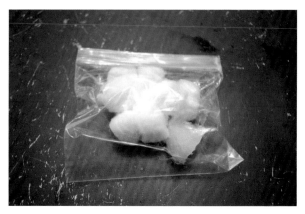

Kneading in a bag is the best way not
to make a mess

1. Scoop some Vaseline into the Ziploc bag (a tablespoon per 4–6 balls seems to work well).
2. Add cotton balls.
3. Knead until well mixed (but don't totally saturate the ball—you will need some dry inner fibers to catch a spark)

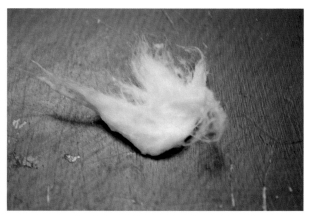

Grease-soaked ball pulls apart and
catches sparks

To use, pull out a ball and gently pull it apart to catch sparks from your keychain firestarting rod—or you can leave whole and light with a match.

A ball made this way should burn for about 4 minutes, giving plenty of time to catch pencil sized and smaller dry twigs on fire.

Type 2—Wax Soaked Lint Balls

Type 2 Materials

Wax soaked lint is a little hard to make, but it burns hotter and longer than the first type. It is better suited for car camping as it is also bulkier and heavier.

Material:

- Dryer lint
- Paraffin wax
- Paper egg carton (not the Styrofoam plastic ones)

Tools:

- Double boiler (or pot and smaller Pyrex measuring cup)
- Scissors

Procedure:

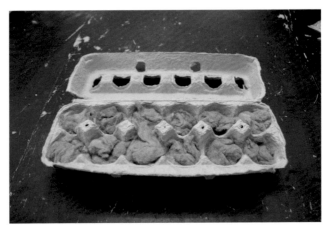

Fill individual egg cartons with dryer lint

1. Fill individual egg cartons with dryer lint.

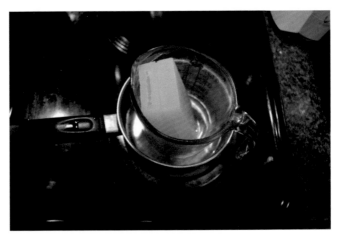

Melt wax in double boiler

2. Melt wax in double boiler by placing wax chunks in the smaller container, placing the smaller container into the larger pot, and then filling the larger pot with boiling water until the level is approximately ⅔ the height of the smaller one.

   2.1. You do not want to get any water in the container holding the wax, and you don't want the water to boil over into the wax pot.

   2.2. The boiling water ensures an even heating so the wax does not overheat and ignite.

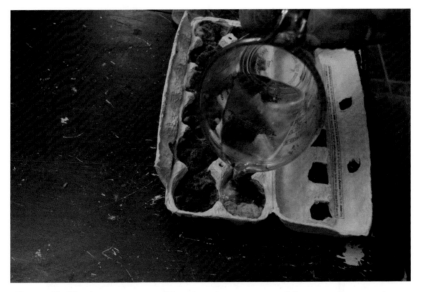

Carefully pour melted wax over the egg carton

3. Carefully pour melted wax over the egg carton until the lint is fully saturated.

4. After the wax cools, cut out the individual egg cartons to make 12 individual fire starters.

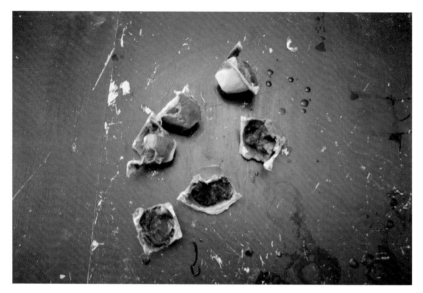

Once wax cools, cut carton into individual
fire starters

Lesson Learned:

Is there a cost difference between the two starters (calculate per unit cost by dividing the cost of the material by number of starters made)? Is there a difference in quality, ease of use, and effectiveness?

This project shows that there are many ways to accomplish the same thing, each with their own strengths and weaknesses, but one is not always better than another.

PROJECT 21

POTATO FANS

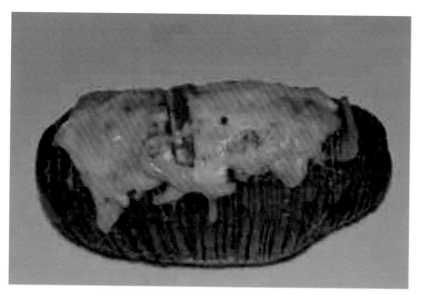

Finished Potato Fan

This is a great recipe for kids, both because it is a simple recipe that most kids can do with a minimum of supervision, but also because it is something most kids will eat. I know I have a toddler who loves them.

From my research into this recipe, I have come to the conclusion that the proper name is probably Hasselback potatoes, since this recipe most likely originated at A Swedish inn named the Hasselbacken.

Since this is nothing more than a fancy baked potato, the best potatoes to use are Russet or Idaho potatoes. I have tried others, but I always get the best result from baking varieties.

Once you get the basic variety down, feel free to add any additional like herbs, crusts, or cheese toppings during the baking process.

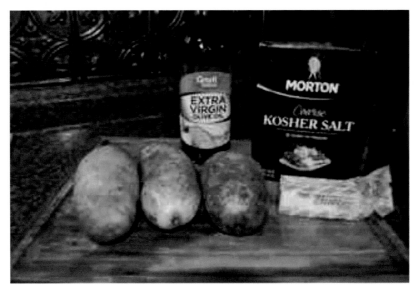

The Basic Ingredients

Ingredients:

- 4 med. potatoes (for best results use uniformly sized oblong potatoes)
- ¼ lb. butter (I normally use a mix of half butter/half oil)
- Coarse Salt

Optional

- ¼ cup cheese
- Herb Blend (¼ teaspoon basil, ¼ teaspoon marjoram, ¼ teaspoon pepper)

Procedure:

1. Preheat oven to 450 degrees F.
2. Oil a large shallow glass baking dish or cookie sheet.

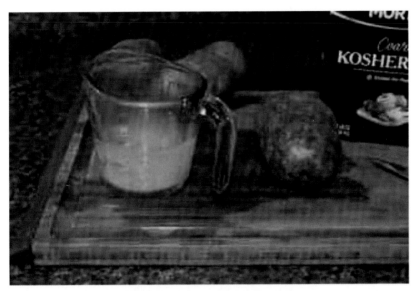

Melted Butter/Oil Mix

3. Melt butter and mix it half/half with olive oil, if desired.
4. Rinse and scrub the potatoes thoroughly.

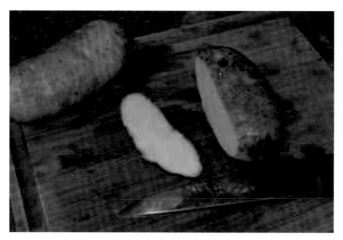

Cut this slice out of potato so it will sit
flat and not roll

5. Cut a thin slice along the long axis of the potato so that
   it will not roll.
6. Place two long handled wooden spoons or other equally
   sized round utensils on either side of the potato (this keeps
   your cuts equal without slicing through the potato).

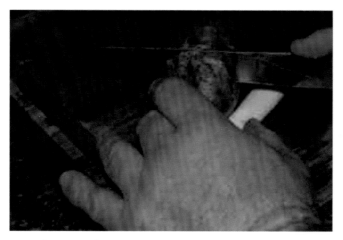

Cut uniform slices without cutting all the way
through the potato

7. Using a sharp knife, slice each potato crosswise into multiple ¼-inch thick slices, cutting down vertically. (the thinner you cut the crispier the finished product)

8. As you finish cutting each potato, drop it into cold water to prevent discoloring.

9. Gently flex the potato fans open while rinsing under cold running water.

10. Dry potatoes well before baking.

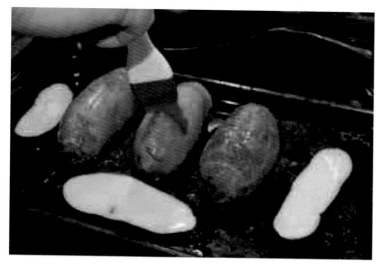

Brush with melted butter/oil mix

11. Brush each potato with butter.

12. Season with salt and herb blend.

13. Place potatoes in the oiled baking dish or cookie sheet and bake 30 minutes.

14. Remove from oven and brush again with oil—at this point add cheese if desired.

15. Return to oven and bake an additional 30 minutes. Potatoes are done when the internal temperature is 200 degrees F.

16. Remove from the oven.
17. Drizzle with remaining melted butter.

Yield:

Serves 4

Lesson Learned:

This is really nothing more than a fancy way to make a baked potato. It is very simple, but it looks fancy, which illustrates that skill can add value.

It also teaches planning, especially if cooking with other items. The first time I made this recipe, I skimmed it and missed the second cooking time and went ahead with my shorter cooking items, which really messed the timing up on my dinner.

Additionally, this is a great recipe for your child to make when dining with others. It is sure to be commented on which will definitely make them feel good about the effort they added to the recipe.

PROJECT 22

BUG OUT BAG

If you are going to participate in personal preparedness, at some point you will want to construct some sort of bag that contains survival essentials. While these bags have numerous names that stem from the intended use, the type of equipment stored, the group that originated them, or the preferences of the owner, the name really doesn't matter.

What matters is that the bag is light and small enough to be portable and contains enough to be useful.

When I was in middle school, I built several survival type bags. I had small belt-sized kits to large backpacks that were pre-packed so I could be prepared in the event of a disaster.

When creating a kit take into consideration the likely threats—i.e., you have no need of a fishing kit if you live in a desert. But also look at your skills. Some people can make fire with natural materials, but others need to ensure their kit has a lighter and matches.

I also like to ensure that I have some sort of entertainment in my bag. For me that means a small novel, but for my young son it may mean a small coloring book and an 8-pack of crayons and lots of diapers . . . .

Material:

- Sturdy kid sized pack
- Depends on the child but you may want to consider:
  - o Medication
  - o Signaling devices (like a cell phone)
  - o Small amounts of cash
  - o Food
  - o Water
  - o First Aid kit
  - o Small knife
  - o Change of clothes
  - o Emergency blanket

Procedure:

1. There is no real procedure to this, simply discuss with your child things they may worry about, look at their personal situation (no taking meds or knives in a school bag), and create a kit that makes you both feel safer without throwing in so much gear that the bag sits in a corner unused.
2. When packing, put items used more often nearer the bag openings.
3. Don't forget to make a kit for each member of your family.
4. Try to ensure you have the essentials to survive 72 hours just on the contents of your kits.

Lessons Learned:

Preplanning is essential to being prepared. But gear alone is not the answer. The more you know and the better you plan and educate yourself the less equipment you can get by on.

PROJECT 23

72 HOUR KIT TEST

This project could well be a part of project 22, however, in my experience one usually forgets about testing a kit when they're focused on building one. Life always interferes and the testing phase always is subject to getting around to it.

By separating the two, I hope that you make the time needed to have a real test of your kit. I am always amazed at how much you learn about your needs when you get around to testing your plans.

Material:
- Family 72 hour kits

Procedure:
1. Pick a weekend that the family can commit to testing the kits. Tell friends and family you will be unavailable for the weekend.

2. If possible, turn off water and power at breaker/water main—otherwise, unplug all devices and commit to not using any utilities.

3. Attempt to last a weekend using only the items in your kits. If you "cheat," make a list of items needed that were not in your kits so you can add them later.

4. It is important that you approach this as a family activity and try to make it as fun as possible.

5. After the experiment is over, take time (after hot showers and a good meal) to have a family discussion of what went well, and what would be needed to make the situation better. Do not allow the family talk to point out personal failings or problems—it should be focused on items and procedures that would make the process easier not events that went wrong.

6. Take what you learned, apply it, and have another test weekend a few months later. After 2 or 3 of these events, you will be surprised at how much easier they become.

Lessons Learned:

The "after action" discussion will shed a lot of light on what is nice and what is needed. Tests like this also show the value of teamwork and family, as well as build confidence.

PROJECT 24

COMPOST PILE

In an earlier project we made seed pots to start seeds, and discussed the need to learn to garden before it became necessary.

This project takes that just a little farther by building a compost bin to make gardening easier.

I live in a subdivision myself, and understand that this is not always practicable due to zoning, but you would be surprised at how many places allow this if done with a little research.

Before you get into composting, you need to realize that a compost pile is an entire ecosystem—it only works because things live in it—you can think of your compost pile as a pet, and like a pet some things are good food, and other things will make it sick. Just like you should not feed your dog chocolate, you should not feed your compost pile meat or fats/oil. It also needs a balanced diet of green plant material and brown vegetation.

Green compost is "wet" things like grass clippings and vegetable peels containing a lot of nitrogen, while brown compost is considered to be "dry" and is full of carbon from dead leaves and sticks.

Your pile needs a 50/50 mix of brown and green, but since green weighs more you should add two or three times the volume of brown for each unit of green that you add.

Typical green materials are:
- Vegetable and fruit scraps
- Coffee grounds and filters
- Tea bags and leaves
- Fresh grass clippings
- Plant trimmings from your garden
- Houseplants

Brown materials are things like:
- Dry leaves
- Straw and dry hay
- Woodchips and sawdust from untreated wood
- Dried grass clippings
- Shredded paper (including newsprint, paper towels, and cardboard)
- Egg and nut shells
- Hair and animal fur

Materials that are bad for your compost pile are:
- Meat
- Fish
- Eggs
- Dairy
- Oily foods or grease
- Bones

- Feces
- Diseased plants and seeds of weedy plants
- Anything treated with pesticides (Remember, your pile is alive)

The smaller you chop your materials, the faster they will break down. You should also be aware that flies may be attracted to some of the greens you put in your pile, so cover them up with a layer of brown. Luckily this also cuts down on any smell.

You should turn your compost at least once a year (more is probably better). I use a pile system where I shovel a pile over to make a new pile to the right of the original mound. I then start a new pile where the original pile was. This ensures that I always have some compost ready to use, and have a pile or two cooking.

A neat side effect of a compost pile is that the decomposition creates heat. I have known people to add a coiled water hose inside the pile to create hot water.

Lesson Learned:

This project is a great opening to discuss biodegradation and why trash needs to be disposed of appropriately, as well as the benefits of reducing, reusing, and recycling.

PROJECT 25

CONTAINER GROWN STRAWBERRIES

Eating food that you have grown yourself is a reward that most modern folks have not had the privilege of having. While most people in today's world can't have huge gardens, I haven't found anyone yet that cannot grow a few plants in containers.

After studying what would be the best container grown plant for this book I settled on strawberries. One reason is that they grow well in indoor containers and only need a sunny spot where they can get 6–8 hours of sunlight. The other reason is that most kids love strawberries, and that once you have one well established plant, it will put out suckers that turn into new plants that you can either grow or give away to your friends.

Before you can grow strawberries in a container, you need to decide what kind of strawberries to grow. Basically there are three types: June-bearing, ever-bearing, or day neutral.

June-bearing strawberries produce a large crop during a three-week period each year.

Ever-bearing strawberries produce two crops of berries, one in the spring and another in the late summer or fall.

Day bearing produces fruit continuously from June through September. However, day neutral strawberries will not flower or bear fruit during hot weather.

Plant your strawberries in the early spring in areas with a cold winter (zones 1 through 5), as soon as the soil can be worked. In warmer areas, strawberries can be planted in the fall.

If you plan to keep them inside, you can plant your strawberries at any time of year.

I like to add a controlled-release fertilizer to the soil before planting in potting soil. Plant your strawberries so the midpoint of the crown is even with the soil's surface and the roots are fanned out.

Water your plants well after planting and check daily. Water frequently until the plants take root; after that, water whenever the top inch of soil is dry.

Strawberries are ready to be picked as soon as the fruit has turned red.

Strawberries can be stored for about two days in shallow trays in the refrigerator. For longer periods, it is best to freeze them. However, I find that when my son and I pick strawberries, they rarely last long enough to make it into the house.

What I like best about strawberries is how easily they reproduce using runners. This means I am able to reproduce new plants at no cost, as well as get new plants with the exact same genes as the plants I choose to propagate.

This is even better because strawberry plants are only productive for three to five years. Aging plants yield smaller and fewer berries, by using runners I can keep myself in new plants without breaking my piggy-bank.

Fall is a good time to cut runners from existing plants and re-plant them to establish new plants. Fall-planted runners will produce a crop the following spring; however, spring-planted runners will not produce berries until the following spring.

The procedure to reproduce your plants using runners is simple:

As the plants grow they put off runners—basically long vines with small leaves at the end—ensure the end of the runner contacts bare soil—it will then start to root. You don't want to bury it though—if it is covered with soil it may rot. I use a bent wire to hold it gently to the ground like a staple

After a few weeks, the runner will root. Cut the stem that connects the runner to its parent plant.

Clip all but two or three of the leaflets from each new little plant.

I then plant the new plant in a new bed—about 6–8 inches from other plants.

Lesson Learned:

Growing food teaches self-reliance and creates a sense of accomplishment. The process of growing something and waiting for results also reinforces self-discipline and patience.

PROJECT 26

PORTABLE DIY FISHING GEAR

Here is a great little PVC fishing pole that has been around for a long time. There are many good videos online that show small PVC fishing kits that are very similar to this one.

I do like having a small lightweight pole that fits in my camping gear so that I can easily dip a line in the water when the opportunity presents itself.

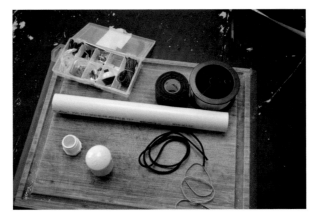

The Materials

Materials:
- ¾-inch MIP PVC plug
- 1 foot of 1-inch diameter schedule 40 PVC pipe
- 1-inch diameter PVC cap
- 18 inches black parachute cord
- 1 roll athletic tape
- 80 feet 10-pound-test fishing line
- 2 thick 1-inch diameter rubber bands
- 3 fishing lures
- 6 size-10 fishing hooks
- 8 size-5 split-shot weights
- Spray paint (optional)

Tools:
- Hacksaw
- Drill with ¼-inch bit

Procedure:
1. If you desire a painted fishing pole, go ahead and paint all the parts now so that they dry before you begin assembly.
2. Insert the ¾-inch MIP PVC plug into one end of the one foot section of PVC pipe.

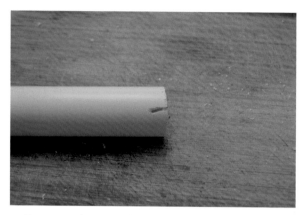

Cut a slit in the end of the pipe

3. At the open end of the PVC pipe, cut a ½ inch long slit into the side of the pipe.
4. Cut a ½ inch long slit into one side of the PVC Pipe cap. Make the slit twice as wide as the saw blade is thick. To do this you may need to cut in angles (make an "X").

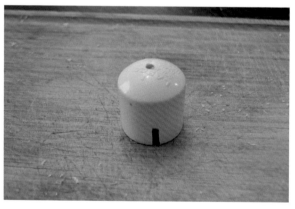

PVC end cap

5. Drill a ¼-inch hole through the top of the cap.
6. Make a loop of parachute cord by tying the ends of the paracord in a knot.

7. Thread the end of the paracord loop through the hole in the cap leaving the knot inside the cap.

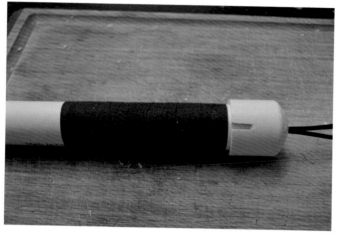

Cap inserted on pole
(with athletic tape in place)

8. Put the cap on the pipe.
9. Starting ¼ inch from the base of the cap, wrap 4 inches of pipe with athletic tape.

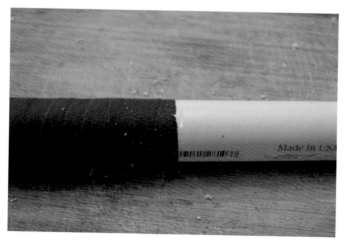

Groove cut in pole

10. Cut a ¹⁄₁₆ inch deep groove across the pipe 4 inches from the plugged end. (10.1. Do not cut through to the inside of the pipe.)

11. Make a few wraps of fishing line around the pipe, ensuring the line rests in the groove cut near the plugged end of the pipe, and then knot tightly.

12. Pull the fishing line toward the plugged end and wrap a 3-inch piece of tape around the pipe to cover the line.

13. Wrap the rest of the fishing line around this piece of tape.

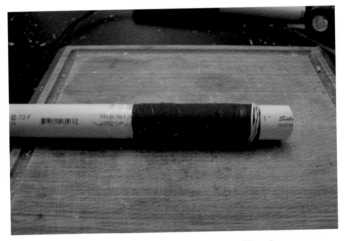

Line and band installed

14. Use rubber bands to hold the wraps of fishing line in place.

15. Tie a favorite lure to the end of the line.

16. Fill the inside of the pipe with fishing supplies, and then place the lure that is tied to the line inside the pipe, ensuring that the line runs out of the slit cut into the end of the pipe.

17. Insert the pipe cap over the end of the pipe, capturing the fishing line in the slit. This keeps the lure securely held.

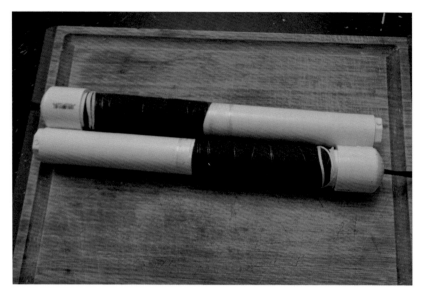

Finished poles—it's just as easy to
make two as one

Usage:

1. Remove the cap and pull out the tied lure.
2. Replace the cap and remove the rubber band holding the wraps of line.
3. Pull approximately one yard of line off the spool and hold the rest of it on with your thumb.
4. Swing the lure over your head in a counterclockwise motion. When you've got it swinging as fast as you can, whip the lure toward the water and take your thumb off the spool. This allows the line to be pulled off in a neat cast.
5. To reel it in, slowly wrap the line around the handle.
6. When you feel the fish bite, give the line a quick jerk to set the hook and reel it in!

Lesson Learned:

Building things exercises special ability, problem solving, and teaches cause and effect.

Anytime you have to measure and drill you are building attention to detail.

Plus you get to go fishing when you are done with this project.

PROJECT 27

WIRE BASKETS

This is a neat project, which makes a useful basket—which you can use to organize or meet some metalworking requirements on a scouting merit badge.

I like them for gardening, as I can easily wash my fruit and vegetables off with the hose before I bring them in the house.

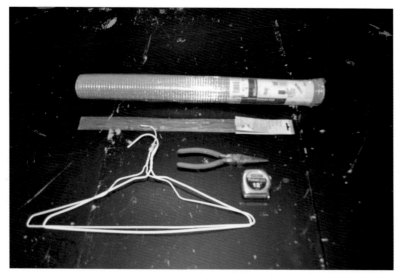

The Materials

Material:
- 2' x 10' Hardware cloth
- 26-gauge Floral wire
- Metal Coat hanger (Optional)
- Rubber hose (Optional)

Tools:
- Tin Snips
- Needle nose pliers

Procedure:
1. When designing your basket you need to allow for the sides. We are going to make a 5-inch deep 8 by 8 inch basket to carry in our vegetables. Since the sides will fold up we will need to cut out a piece of wire that is 18 inches square.

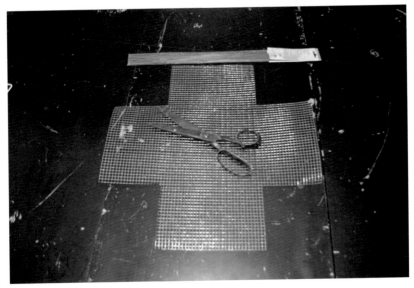

Screen cut into a cross shape

2. Using tin snips cut this into a cross shape with 5 inch squares taken out of each corner. This will make eight inch "wings" that stick out on each of the 4 sides.

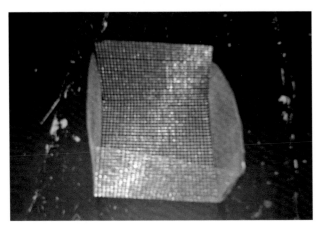

Fold into a box shape

3. Make your creases/folds along the "wings."
4. Cut the floral wire 1.5x the size of the side you're going to connect. This means for a 5 inch seam, cut the wire 7.5 inches (or 8 if you want extra).

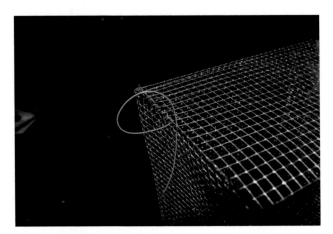

Thread wire to sew edges

5. Start at one end, and pull the wire almost all the way through leaving about 1" of slack to wrap around that first corner several times before weaving up the side. (5.1. Hitting every square looks better, and makes a stronger basket, but you can save time by only weaving every other square if you desire.)

6. Lastly, trim the ends of your wire, and tidy up the basket.

7. If you desire you can make handles by cutting up a metal coat hanger and using needle nose pliers to create loops on each end

8. You can make the handle fit your hand better by sliding a rubber hose (like an aquarium hose) over the coat hanger before attaching it to the basket.

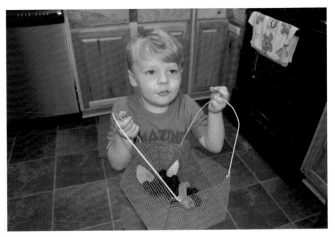

Basket full of growies

Lesson Learned:

This is a great geometry starter; looking at how a flat surface can be made into a three dimensional object can be really intriguing for someone with an active imagination. This is a cheap project so it lends itself to experimentation.

PROJECT 28

KITCHEN SCRAP GARDENING

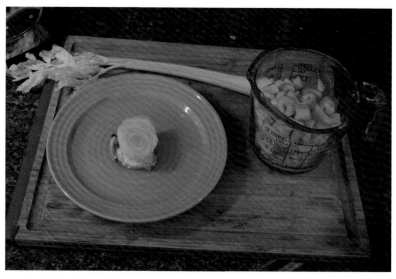

Celery Stalk

A nifty beginning gardening trick is gardening by planting kitchen scraps. It is possible to have everlasting celery by replanting scraps from your harvested celery stalk.

When I tried this for the first time I was amazed at how easy and forgiving this process is. This makes it perfect for kids to do in the kitchen.

Material:
- Celery stalk
- Water

Tools:
- Knife
- Saucer
- Sunny window

Procedure:
1. After cutting up celery for any recipe take the base of the stalk and set it in a saucer filled with some water.
2. Set the saucer in a sunny area of your kitchen and over the next couple of weeks check it every couple of days to ensure that the saucer still has some water in it.
3. The celery will sprout and then you can either plant it in your garden, or in a container indoors.

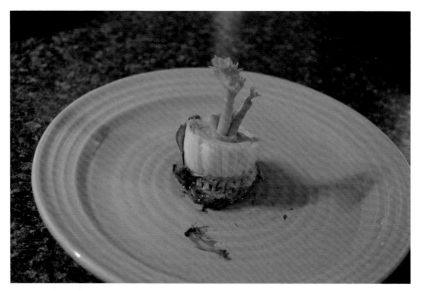

Celery growing from discarded stalk

4. When the celery grows big enough, harvest your free celery and replant the cut end for an endless supply of home raised vegetables.

Lesson Learned:

This is a great opportunity to talk about recycling and reusing items to prevent waste.

PROJECT 29

PIE IRON PIZZA

This is a fun "camping" recipe that kids of a vast range of ages can make themselves with little adult supervision.

While being a easy favorite for kids, it is also infinitely adaptable. You can use it with eggs and sausage to make a breakfast meal, eat it for lunch or dinner, use pizza dough, biscuit dough, or sliced bread—or even use apples and sugar to make it a dessert.

As with many of my projects, once you learn the technique you can take it and make it your own special recipe.

Material:
- 2 pieces of bread per pizza
- Butter
- Pizza Sauce
- Shredded Cheese
- Dried Italian Seasoning (Oregano)
- Garlic Salt

- Toppings
  - pepperoni, pre-cooked sausage, hamburger, whatever you want—or just make a cheese pizza

Tools:

- Pie iron (Unless it's just for one or two people, one pie iron is never enough.)
- Campfire gloves
- Knife
- Spatula

Procedure:

1. Heavily butter one side of each piece of bread.
    1.1. For biscuit dough and pizza crust dough—heavily butter the pie iron instead.
    1.2. Pull biscuit dough until it is flattened out to fit the inside of the pie iron—use 1 biscuit for each side
    1.3. For pizza crust: butter the pie iron, lay the dough inside one half of the pie iron with an equal portion hanging over, then fold the back over the toppings before closing pie iron.

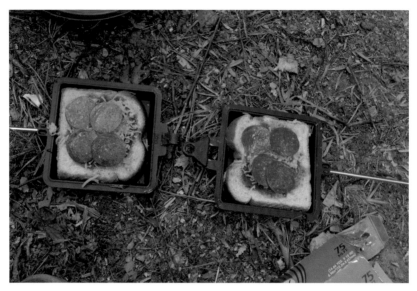

Put toppings on a generously
buttered slice of bread

2. Generously spread pizza sauce on one side of bread/bis-cuit/dough—to suit your taste.

3. Add shredded cheese, and toppings if used.

4. Spread pizza sauce on the other piece of bread/biscuit, or flap of pizza crust.

5. Season with oregano and garlic salt, then close pie iron.

6. For pizza crust—fold flap in, over cheese and toppings first.

7. Trim off any excess ingredients sticking out of the closed iron.

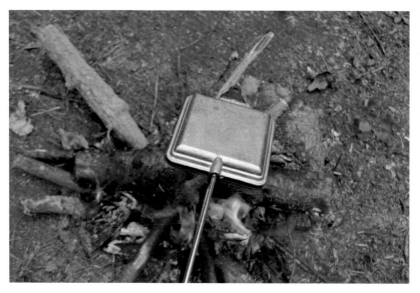

Cook over coals

8. Cook over medium coals, or low campfire flame.

    8.1. For bread pizza: after three minutes, rotate pie iron and cook for four more minutes.

    8.2. For biscuit and pizza dough: rotate after four minutes, and cook for five more minutes

    8.3. These are only approximate times. Use your own judgment and keep in mind that pie irons can be closed and pizzas re-cooked if you want them more well-done, but you cannot "un burn" pizza.

9. Open pie irons and use a spatula to remove pizza.

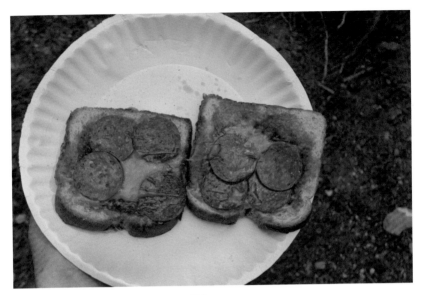

Pizza

CAUTION! Pie irons will be very hot, and the insides of the just-cooked pizza will be very hot! Do not let young kids try to handle them until they have time to cool—which should only be a few minutes.

Lesson Learned:

This is a fun way to learn that sometimes there are many ways to get similar results. This in turn creates flexibility, adaptability, and understanding.

PROJECT 30

TIN CAN LANTERN

This is a simple project that is a flexible way to make light. This project works well with the lint fire starters, bottle cap candles, tea lights, or even a large gob of shortening as a candle fuel.

Care must be taken with the fuel used to ensure that it does not fall out of the lantern and start a fire. You need to be aware of the sharp edges present in the aluminum can.

The idea to use a discarded metal container to make a light is not new; pioneers have done this with tin cans for decades. The metal has changed, but not the idea.

Material
- Aluminum can
- Wire
- Candle

Tools
- Knife or Scissors
- Marker

Procedure

1. Rinse out a empty aluminum can and let dry.
2. Turn empty can on its side and draw a large "H" on the can.
   2.1. The sides of the "H" should be no larger than ⅓ the diameter of the can
   2.2. The inside line connecting the sides of the "H" should be approximately 1 inch from the top and bottom of the can.
3. Carefully cut along the marked lines of the "H."
4. Taking care not to get cut on the sharp edges, gently fold the cut areas out so you can see inside the can.
5. Use a wire tied to the pop top on the lid of the can to create a handing loop.
6. Insert a candle.

Be careful to ensure that the lantern is hung in an area free of combustibles. It will get hot, so do not leave it burning unattended.

Lesson Learned:

Recycling is great, but reusing is better. Taking trash and using skill and imagination to make something useful is a great way to create value.

PROJECT 31

BOOK CODE

Kids love codes. Playing spy is fun, but it can also be educational. The book code is an easy introduction to cryptology and can cultivate an interest in higher-level math skills.

It is also an easy way to leave a private message for the family in the event of a major disaster. If your child finds this book code interesting, it may pay to research dead drops, code words, and other useful ideas from the "spy" world.

Material:
- Two copies of the same book—they must be identical. I like to use mass market fiction paperbacks—just about any used book store will carry the exact same versions of paperback authors like Stephen King, Dean Koontz, trade westerns, or (not for kids) romance novels . . . .
- Paper and Pen

Procedure:

1. Decide what book you will use as a code and share it with your partner.

2. Create a short message like "I went to town, will be back at 2 p.m."

3. Take each word of your message and find that word somewhere in your book.

4. For each word write down the page number, line number, and word number.

   4.1. Example: a word on page 7, third line down, fifth word would become 7.3.5, or something similar depending on the method you devise.

   4.2. Using the first paperback printing of the book *52 Unique Techniques for Stocking Food for Preppers*, the code 19-1-1 101-1-3 4-25-9 translates to "This is fun."

Remember to always use the SAME version of the book, not just the same book

This is not a foolproof code; today's computers can easily break book codes, but it is fun to experiment with secret codes.

For a more foolproof code, come up with predetermined code words that can be encrypted into a book code (or conversation) for instance "I am going on vacation" could mean "I went to grandma's house."

Lesson Learned:

Learning critical thinking skills, observation, and self-discipline is not always easy, but this project introduces these concepts in a fun way.

Cryptology opens doors to higher level math, and some understanding of codes is vital to learning computer science.

PROJECT 32

PARACORD BRACELET

Weaving paracord seems to be a perennial favorite of scout-aged children. When I was a young teenager on staff at my local scout camp it was popular, and from YouTube videos I see it still is.

I have known enterprising young men and women make spending money from weaving paracord bracelets and other useful items.

Woven paracord rifle slings are very popular in the prepping and wilderness survival groups because it is a useful way to carry a significant amount of cordage. I myself have woven a handle on the bag I carry to work for just this reason.

Once the basics are mastered, all manner of variations can be created.

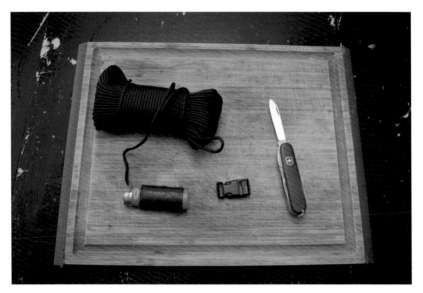

The Materials

Material:

- Approximately 10 feet of paracord (or similar ⅛" diameter string) (1 foot of cord for every 1 inch of knotted length.)
- Side release buckle

Tools:

- Tape measure or ruler
- Scissors
- Lighter

Procedure:

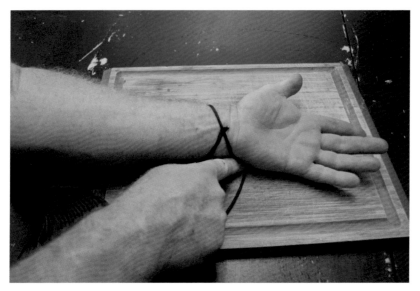

Measure your wrist

1. Measure your wrist by wrapping the paracord around your wrist and mark where the cord meets.
2. The distance between marks is your wrist size. You will need a little more than 1 foot of cord per inch of wrist size (remember to leave a little extra)
3. Find the center of the cord you will be using by holding the ends of the cord together and stretching it to make a loop.
4. Pull the loop through one end of the buckle.

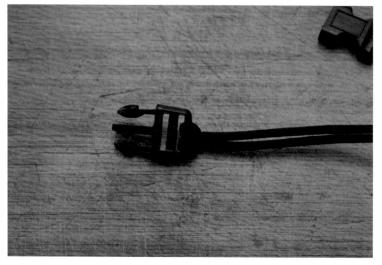

Loop cord through buckle

5. Pull the cord ends thru the loop until it's tightened up and attached to the buckle.
6. Take buckle apart and pull the free ends of the rope through the other half of the buckle.

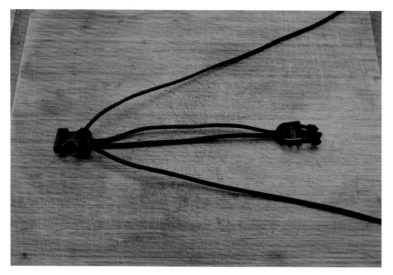

Bring the cord through both buckle ends

7. Add one inch to your wrist measurement (to ensure a comfortable fit) and slide the free end of the buckle down the paracord until you have that distance between the two buckle ends.

   7.1. Remember that the buckle counts in the total wrist measurement, but that the prongs on the male end of the buckle don't count as they will be inside the female half of the buckle.

8. Now you are ready to start knotting. The knot used is called a Portuguese sinnet, a cobra stitch, or a Solomon bar.

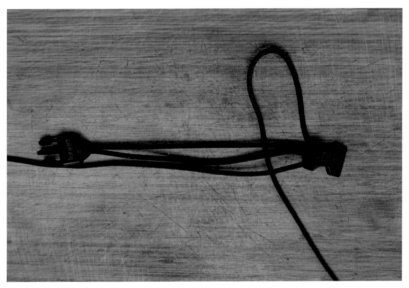

Start weaving from the left

9. Starting with the buckle end that is free, take the cord on the left side and place it under the two center strands.

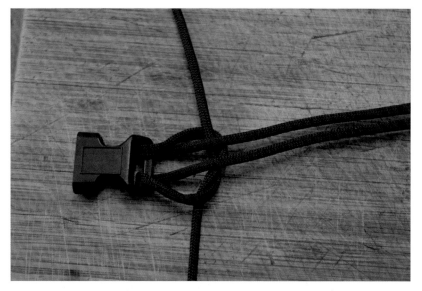

Once tightened this is one complete knot

10. Take the cord on the right side, move it under the end of the left side cord, slide it over the two center strands, and through the loop on the left side.
11. Tighten the string until it is snug (but not collapsed) against the buckle.
12. Take the right side under the two center strands, and then pull the left side cord around it, over the center two cords, and then loop around the right side cord.
13. Tighten this and you will have a completed knot.

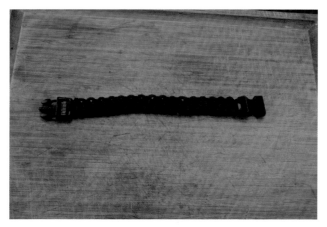

Alternating knots keep the braid flat

14. Continue alternating left to right and tighten as you go.
    14.1. If you do not alternate the knot will twist. If it does so, just undo the last knots until it corrects itself.
15. Keep the knots uniformly tightened with the same tension and size.
16. When the knots get to the buckle end, trim the ends closely and melt the ends.

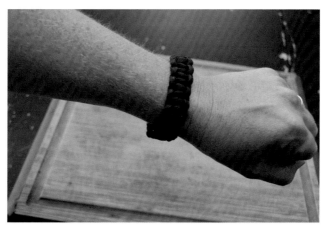

Finished bracelet

Lesson Learned:

This is a great way for a budding entrepreneur to make some pocket money. Be sure to calculate the cost of materials, time, and other costs to calculate a break even price.

PROJECT 33

PREPPER GAMES

The goal of preparedness is to reduce fear—not CAUSE it. A central tenet of my family life is that preparedness should be a family activity. It should make life easier and sometimes it makes life more fun.

Making games out of learning causes skill acquisition to be fun, which means kids will actively participate in things that may save their life one day.

Here are a few such games:

Go on a Picnic—Without notice, grab your "go bag" or 72 hour kit and head outside. Go to the park or local forest and have a picnic. Do you have enough water, food, and other items to do so comfortably? What things would you and your kids add to make it easier? Take what you learn and add to your kit. Repeat as necessary and eventually it will become habit—what better way to spend time and build skills than picnicking with the family?

Lights Out—In order to make the darkness less scary, ensure everyone knows the power outage plan and where the flashlights are, turn the lights out one evening, and cook dinner using alternative methods. After the meal, enjoy family activities by flashlight (no ghost stories). Pop popcorn, talk about the pioneers, read by firelight, and sleep in sleeping bags in the living room.

Sleeping Out—Once the family is used to the dark by playing Lights out, take it up a notch by camping outside. Practice cooking over a campfire by using a grill if you can't build a proper campfire. As the family gains skill, start reducing the amount of creature comforts.

Hide and Seek—Kids love hide and seek because they get the thrill of being chased as well as having the opportunity to outsmart the "hunter." In the preparedness version, first teach the kids where the safe spots are. In our home, by practicing this game, we learned that the place we had designated as a safe spot for our child to hide was actually in the line of fire in any defensive shooting situation. This game helps reinforce where to hide if there is an intruder, as well as help parents know where their kids may hide when scared. From working many missing child searches, I have learned that most kids are found in or near the home.

Road Trip—With no notice, have everyone pack what they need for an extended road trip—no destination given and only fifteen minutes to be packed and in the car. Reward the effort with a road trip to somewhere cool—like a state park. However, the family can only use what they packed—over time, the packing will be quicker, neater, and things will not be forgotten as often.

Where's Home?—Another great skill is to randomly quiz your kids about where they are and how to get home from where they are. A form of this exercise is done quite often with police or fire service rookies to teach situational awareness.

Where Am I?—While free-range parenting is not always in style, knowing where your kids are is always helpful. Keep a map on the fridge and let the kids mark where they are going to be playing. A simple drawing of the house and backyard works great for smaller kids, while older kids can use more sophisticated maps. This allows for some level of freedom as well as a sense of responsibility. Of course, there has to be consequences for not being in the areas marked.

Scavenger Hunt—A popular game I played at scout meetings was "find the penny," where older scouts hid small objects in a fixed area and we tried to find them. This taught observation skills as well as gave the adults time to get some work done.

Playing Doctor—One of the games I played as a kid that helped develop my ability to adapt items to fit needs outside of the items original design was playing doctor. My scout troop spent a lot of time "fixing" broken legs, arms, collarbones and all manner of other injuries by adapting magazines, coat hangers, bandannas and other items into splints.

Kim's Game—In Rudyard Kipling's *Kim*, Kim was trained as a spy by playing a game in which he was shown a tray of jewels, given the opportunity to handle, count, and memorize the contents, then have it covered and being asked to write down the contents from memory. The USMC sniper instructor school uses this to teach observation and it is a game that even preschool children can play.

Drawing—Another common tool taught in military sniper schools is to draw detailed pictures of an area under observation. By having kids draw what they see you can teach them to see and observe and not just look.

Lessons Learned:

Each game teaches a slightly different skill, and over time they become more advanced. Games make practice seem fun and less like the valuable work that they are. These games teach observation, adaptability, navigation, situational awareness, the ability to organize and think ahead, and to become comfortable dealing outside of their comfort zone.

PROJECT 34

SOLAR AUTO SHADE REFLECTOR OVEN

I have made several solar ovens, some being overly complex, others being ineffective, but when I saw this simple solar reflector oven made from an auto shade I found it to be perfect for introduction the concept.

It is simple, cheap, and it works.

While it is flimsy, and you may need to use sticks to hold it in place in windy weather, the material allows for it to be tilted toward the sun, or be folded up and stored easily.

Temperatures of 350 degrees F can easily be reached.

Material:
- Reflective accordion-folding car sunshade
- Bucket or cardboard box
- Cake rack, wire frame, or grill grate (optional)
- Black Pot
- Oven cooking bag

Tools:
- Scissors
- Tape

Procedure:
1. Place a black pot on top of a square cake rack.
2. Put the pot and rack inside a plastic baking bag.
3. Place the rack on the tope of the bucket.
4. Lay the sunshade out.
5. Bring the edges together and tape into a funnel shape around the pot.
   - 5.1. Since the shade is flexible it needs to sit on the wire rack.
   - 5.2. It also allows the sun's rays to reflect on all sides of the pot.

Lessons Learned:
This project is a great way to learn that solar energy is more useful that just using solar panels to make electricity. It is actually a much more efficient use of the sun to make heat rather than convert to electricity, then convert the electricity to chemical energy (batteries), back to electricity, then to work (causing heat).

48 HOUR CANDLE

Being able to have light in the dark is an essential disaster skill. It is more than being able to see, but also for the emotional comfort.

This project is simple, cheap, and versatile. If you need more light, add more wicks to the tub of shortening. If you need light for a longer time, use fewer wicks.

You can use almost any natural fiber as a wick. Cotton string works best, but rolled up paper towels work in a pinch.

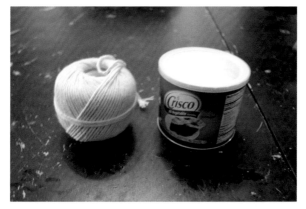

The Materials

Material:

- Tub of shortening
- Cotton string

Procedure:

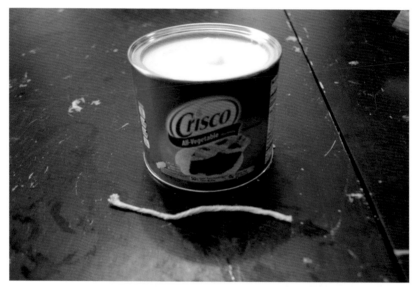

Cut a length of string that is about
as long as the tub is high

1. Cut a length of string that is about as long as the tub is high.
2. Push the string into the tub leaving approximately 1 inch sticking out.

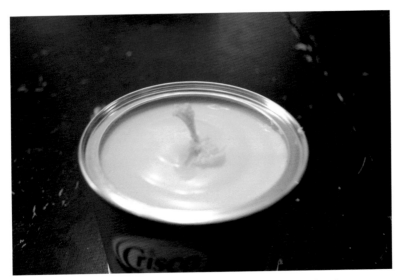

Insert as many wicks as needed
into shortening

3. Light the string.
4. This project requires supervision. Do not leave the candle unattended or it may cause a fire.

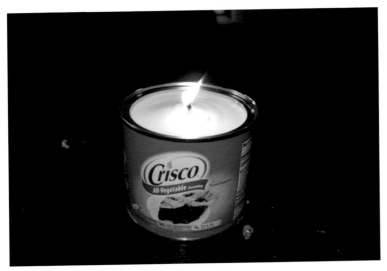

Do not leave candle unattended

Lessons Learned:

Experimenting with multiple wicks reinforces efficiency and the idea of trade offs. More light means less candle time. More time means a lower flame.

PROJECT 36

WATERPROOFING MATCHES

Matches are an easy way to make fire, but wet matches are useless, and since anything worth doing is worth having a redundant method, we are going to show two easy ways to keep your matches dry. One is traditional and uses wax, and the other is easier and uses fingernail polish.

Material:
- Matches
- Candles / Block of Paraffin Wax
- Clear Fingernail Polish
- Newspaper or a piece of cardboard

Tools:
- Double Boiler

Procedure Method 1:

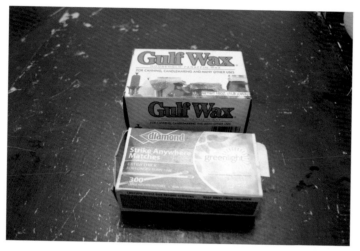

Materials for Wax Method

1. Melt the wax. If you have a candle in a jar, you can melt the wax by burning the candle and then blowing it out, but melting a block of wax in a double boiler is more efficient.

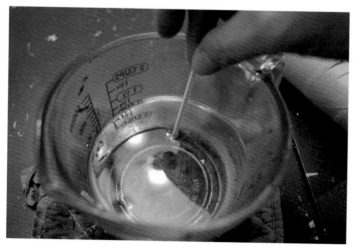

Dip into wax

2.   Dip your matches in the melted wax

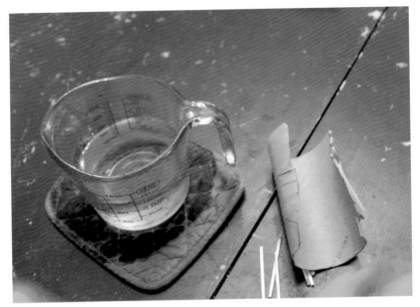

Cool on cardboard

3.   Let the individual matches cool on some newspaper or cardboard to catch drips.

4.   To use these matches you need to scrape the wax off the tip with your fingernail. You also need to store them in a way that keeps the wax from rubbing off due to excessive movement.

Procedure Method 2:

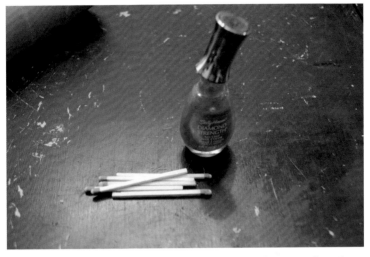

Materials for fingernail polish method

1. Paint the match heads with fingernail polish. (1.1. They need to be thoroughly covered, but not globbed over excessively.)

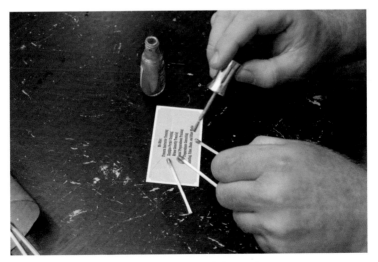

Brush on and let dry

2. Let the matches dry. This takes little longer to dry than the waxed matches.
3. The good thing about fingernail polish matches is that they don't need any special treatment once dried.

Lessons Learned:

From the earlier projects it is pretty obvious that fire is one of the key skills to learn if a person wants to be independent.

It's not just about what to do with the fire, or even how to build a fire, but also part of the lesson is being prepared to make a fire.

PROJECT 37

MINI SURVIVAL KIT

When I was a child, I used to make little survival kits all the time. It got to the point where my mother could not keep bullion cubes in the house, because every time I saw a container of them I "requisitioned" them to make another survival kit.

As I grew older I became less enamored with survival kits, because I felt they either did not have enough tools to be useful, or—on a slightly different note—I had enough skills where didn't need them.

Now, I have reached a point where I welcome the safety net a well thought out kit brings, as well as confident enough in the use of all the materials I keep in my kit.

When making a kit, take care to plan for the area you operate in, as tools and equipment perfect for a tropical environment would be near useless in a desert. Also think about the skill level of the people using the kit, and the space and size requirements.

A kit perfect for a car is probably too bulky for most to carry on a day hike. Remember, a kit is no good if it is left behind.

This project is geared toward making a more general small pocket kit for temperate climate areas. While the materials listed below are a good start, feel free to modify based upon your needs.

The perfect time to go over basic survival strategies is while making a survival kit. In today's world, rescue won't take more than a day or two if the lost individual is smart and stays in one place and makes themselves easy to find.

Food is not as important as protection from the elements, clean water, and some way to signal.

Material:

- Altoids Tin
  - o Used as a storage container, as well as the body of a solid fuel stove (with the Vaseline cotton balls or commercial fuel tabs).
- 2 Razor Blades
  - o Used to cut string and field dress any game.
- 1 Box Matches
  - o Store in a waterproof container (and waterproof per project 36).
- 4 Cotton Balls with Vaseline in them
  - o These firestarters are described in project 20. ensure you dry and compact them before you place them in the kit.
- 10 Feet Parachute Cord
  - o True paracord has inner threads that can be removed to use as additional cordage.
- 10–20 Feet Snare Wire (Thin Steel Wire)
  - o The wire can be used for shelter construction, but snares are the easiest way to catch game in a survival situation.

Mini Survival Kit

- 20 Feet of Fishing Line
- 6 Medium Size Fishing Hooks
  - Large hooks are next to useless when catching fish for survival.
- 6 Lead Fishing Weights
  - Lead reusable split shot work best.
- Small LED Flashlight
  - I keep a small button LED light on my keychain also.
- Plastic Wrap or plastic sheet
  - A sheet can help in shelter construction, but it is also useful in getting water (see project 46).
- Garbage bags
  - Both for water collection, but also as a raincoat, and to sleep on. Garbage bags are very useful for those that are creative.
- 2 Tylenol/Advil (Vacuum Packed)
  - I also like to keep some Benadryl tablets if space allows.
- 2 Feet Duct Tape
  - I keep a lot of duct tape in my gear (project 6), as it can be used in multiple ways.
- 4–7 Various Sized Safety Pins
- 2 Feet Length of Heavy Duty Aluminum Foil
  - This has some limited use as a reflector for signaling, but it is highly useful for cooking. It can even be folded up to make a cooking pot of sorts.
- Water Purification Tablets
- Tea Bag
- Button Compass
  - "Hug a Tree" and stay where you are is the best survival strategy for kids, but a navigation aid may come in useful.

Tools:

- Sponge
- Acetone
- Soap

Procedure:

1. Remove the paint from the outside of the container by using the acetone and a sponge to rub off the paint.
2. Use soap and water to wash out the inside of the container, otherwise sugar remnants can attract bugs or feed mold.
3. Tightly fold the aluminum foil until it fits easily into the bottom of the container.
4. Fold the garbage bag the same size as the foil using tape to secure the folds. (Place the bag on top of the foil.)
5. Insert the tea bag.
6. Wrap a wide and thin amount of duct tape around your fingers, then place inside the tin.
7. Fit the other items in wherever they fit.
8. Close the tin.
9. Wrap the parachute cord around the outside of the tin

Lessons Learned:

Self-reliance builds confidence.

When talking about wilderness survival with children, stress that no matter how scared they may become, staying in one spot makes it much easier for them to be found.

PROJECT 38

SODA BOTTLE ANTI-DRIP COOLER

I found this idea on Pinterest, and saw how easy it was to do.

Not only is it easy to do, but it serves the purpose of keeping drips contained if you serve juice or Kool-Aid in a push spout cooler.

I like keeping a container of sports drink when we are working out on our land, and drips from the cooler can attract flies and other bugs.

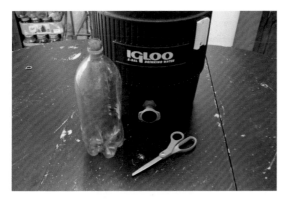

The Materials

Material:

- 2 liter plastic bottle

Tools:

- Scissors

Procedure:

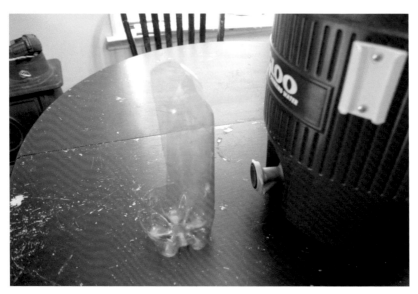

Cut the bottle into an "L" shape

1. Cut the top off of a plastic soda bottle.
2. Cut down and leave an "L" shape at the bottom.
3. Cut a small hole in the top large enough to hang over the spigot of a drink cooler.

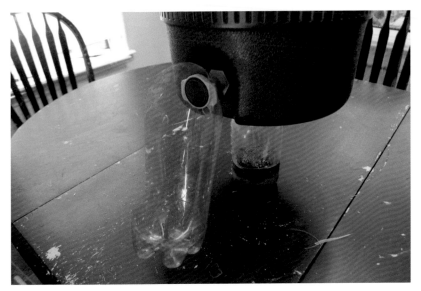

Hang from cooler spigot to catch drips

Lessons Learned:

Besides the hand eye coordination of cutting (for smaller kids), this project enforces the mindset of reduce, reuse, recycle as it uses trash to make something useful.

PROJECT 39

DEHYDRATED FRUIT LEATHER

Commercial fruit leather is pretty popular, and I remember eating "fruit roll ups" as a child. Unfortunately, commercial fruit leathers can be expensive and they can also contain a lot of unnatural additives.

Homemade fruit leathers should not contain anything other than fruit, lemon juice, and MAYBE some sugar (however, we will give some additional options later).

I find that the following fruits work well for fruit leathers, but personal taste may vary:

Apple, apricot, banana, blackberry, blueberry, cherry, cranberry, grapefruit, grape, kiwi, lemon, nectarine, orange, peach, pear, persimmon, pineapple, plum, pumpkin, raspberry, rhubarb, strawberry, watermelon.

Basically you are going to make a sauce with blended fruit and then dehydrate it—so it is possible to use vegetables if you want to get creative.

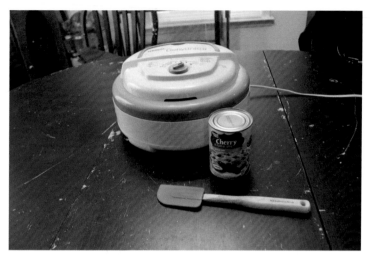

The Materials

Material:

- Fruit
- Lemon juice (to prevent browning)
- Optional sweeteners/flavorings:
  - Fruit juice
  - Honey
  - Maple syrup
  - Brown sugar
  - Fruit jams/preserves
  - Vanilla or almond extract
  - Brandy
  - Cinnamon
  - Nutmeg
  - Ginger

Tools:

- Fruit Peeler
- Blender or Food Mill

- Teaspoon
- Mixing bowl
- Dehydrator
- Solid tray or fruit leather tray

Procedure:

1. Wash fruit and remove cores or large seeds.
2. Peel if desired, but you can also leave the skin on fruits with edible skins.
3. Cut fruit into small pieces and place in a blender.
4. Add a teaspoon of lemon juice to cover the cut fruit to prevent browning from oxygenation.
5. Add any sweetener and flavor you want but don't use too much as it will thin out your mix and make it take a lot of time to dry. Also, some flavorings will cause the dried leathers to be sticky. It is also important to know that dehydrating intensifies flavors so use additions sparingly.
6. Blend until smooth.

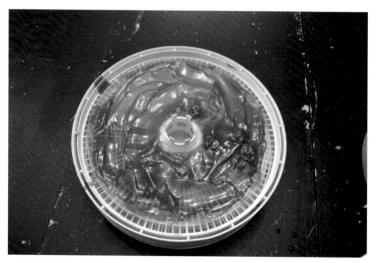

Fruit puree spread on dehydrator sheet

7. Spread parchment paper, Excalibur ParaFlexx, or fruit leather inserts on your dehydrator tray—don't use wax paper.

8. Spread your mix about ⅛-inch thick on your dehydrator tray, but since the edges will dry quicker try to make the edges thicker so that the leather dries evenly.

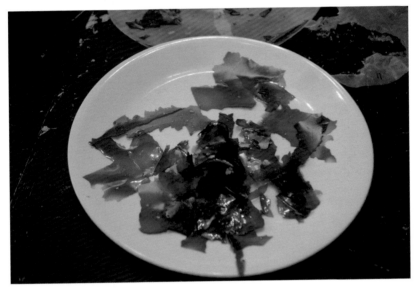

Dried leather peeled off—the thicker, the easier to peel, but the longer the process will take.

9. Set your dehydrator to 135 degrees F.
    9.1. Drying times will usually be in between six to twelve hours; it mostly depends on the water content of your fruit leather.
    9.2. After about six hours, your leather may be dry enough to peel off and place directly on the mesh trays. This will speed up drying.

9.3.   Leather will be pliable not crispy when done. Be sure to check spots where the mixture was spread thicker to make sure there is no moisture.

This is best stored in the refrigerator at home, but wrapped in plastic it can last a few days for use camping or hiking.

If you want, you can add a little water and rehydrate it back into a sauce, but I like to eat it dry.

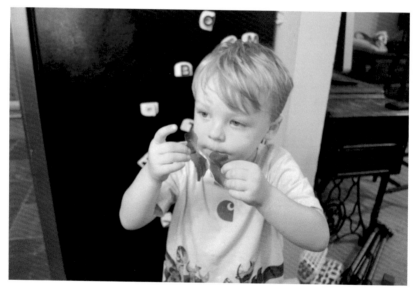

It tastes good

Lessons Learned:

Cooking teaches cause and effect, and by using the dehydrator kids learn patience, as well as how to preserve food using one of the basic food storage methods.

This is also a great way to teach economics as you can compare the cost and quality of homemade fruit leathers with store bought kinds.

PROJECT 40

HOMEMADE LIQUID DISH SOAP

Homemade cleaning products are great because they typically are much cheaper (dramatically so), contain fewer harsh ingredients, and are fun to make.

In other books we have made bar soap, clothes washing soap, and now we focus on dish soap.

By letting our three-year-old splash and play with soapy water and "dirty" dishes we are trying to teach that chores can be fun.

Can you think of a better way to introduce this than by making the soap from scratch?

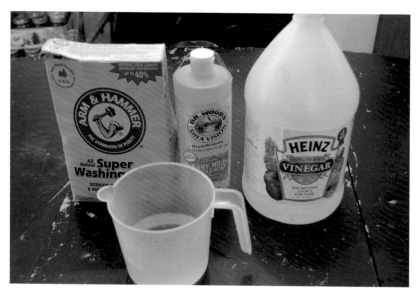

The Ingredients

Material:

- 1 ½ cups of hot water
- ½ cup liquid castile soap
- 1 tablespoon of white vinegar
- 1 tablespoon of washing soda
- ⅛ teaspoon of tea tree oil (optional)

Tools:

- Measuring cups
- Whisk/Mixing spoon
- Large bowl
- Reused Dish Soap dispenser
- Funnel

Procedure:

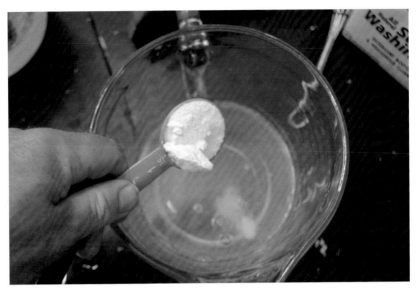

Combine all ingredients and
whisk until combined

1. Combine all ingredients into a large bowl.
2. Pour in 1 ½ cups of very hot water.
3. Whisk/stir this mixture until all ingredients are thoroughly blended and soap has completely melted.
4. ⅛ teaspoon of tea tree oil will increase the antibacterial properties of the soap.
5. Allow mixture to cool completely on the counter.
6. Stir occasionally.

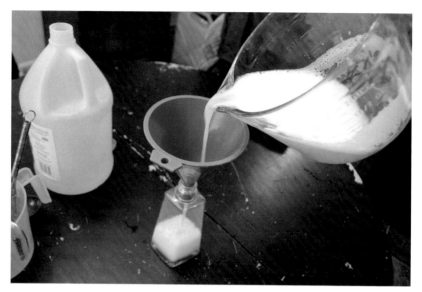

Fill recycled bottle with soap mix

7. Use a funnel to pour the mix into a saved soap dispensing bottle and use as you would commercial soap.

Lessons Learned:

This project is a great beginning household chemistry experiment, and opens the door to great conversations about hygiene, bacteria and germs, and the benefit of learning how to DIY.

PROJECT 41

STRAWBERRY BREAD

If you have ever had banana or zucchini bread you are familiar with the concept behind today's project.

Strawberry bread is a great way to start baking, as it is easy, tasty, and fun.

If you want to bake it with nuts, follow the recipe, but feel free to omit them. Or, you can substitute them if you want. The recipe calls for pecans, but walnuts work well also.

However you choose to make strawberry bread, you can rest assured, it is an easy recipe to try for beginning bakers, and because it tastes good, it is a perfect reinforcement for the joy of cooking.

Ingredients:
- 3 cups flour
- 2 cups white sugar
- 1 teaspoon ground cinnamon
- 1 teaspoon salt
- 1 teaspoon baking soda
- 4 eggs

- 1 ¼ cups vegetable oil
- 1 cup chopped pecans
- 2 ½ cups freeze-dried strawberry slices
- grease

Tools:

- 9" x 5" pan
- Large bowl
- Small bowl
- Spoon
- Mixing cups

Procedure:

1. Preheat oven to 350 degrees F.
2. Grease and flour 9" x 5" pan.
3. In a large bowl, sift together sugar, flour, cinnamon, salt, and baking soda.
4. In a smaller bowl, beat eggs and oil.
5. Stir nuts and strawberries into the egg mix.
6. Add egg mixture to the sifted ingredients and stir until combined.
7. Pour into 9" x 5" pan.
8. Bake for 1 hour or until toothpick inserted in center comes out clean.
9. Let cool and serve.

Lessons Learned:

As with all cooking recipes, this teaches and reinforces cause and effect, basic math, and encourages creativity.

PROJECT 42

SUN HOSE WATER HEATER

This project is an experiment in solar water heating.

Most preppers, homesteaders, and anyone else interested in sustainability or living more ecologically minded are enthusiastic about solar energy. In my experience, solar is much more efficient and easier utilized when it is used for heat rather than electricity.

This is because of the efficiency losses when transferring one type of energy to another (as we discussed in project 34).

Absorbing the sun's heat and using the heat directly is the easiest way to use solar power, and by using solar heat for water, we save energy (either electric or fossil fuels) by not having to run a water heater.

It is possible to construct a solar water heater that is plumbed directly into a home's water system to either pre-heat the water going into the water heater, or to replace it.

This system is better used to wash dirty hands and feet before going back in the house, a dirty dog, or a pre-swim rinse than to use as an actual shower, but I have used this at the land to get a hot shower after a hard day of camping and building.

Material:
- 100–200 feet of garden hose (black is best)
- Sheet of clear plastic or tempered glass (optional)
- Sheet of black plastic (optional)

Procedure:
1. Locate a spot in full sun that won't be bothered; many people choose to put solar water heaters on their roofs, but for this project we will stick with ground level.
2. For best results lay out a sheet of black plastic for the hose to sit on. This will help absorb the heat from the sun.
3. Lay out the hose on the plastic (or straight on the ground). Depending on use, available light, and how quickly you need the water, some layouts work better than others. Experiment with a spiral coil and a back and forth zig-zag pattern. These are the most typical ways to lay out the hose.
4. To weigh down the hose, as well as to help trap the heat, cover the hose with a a piece of tempered glass or plastic if you have one available.

One hundred feet of black hose will heat up in about thirty minutes, and will give enough warm water to for a quick shower. Two hundred feet will allow for a more "normal" shower time.

Be careful though, in the full sun of a hot summer afternoon, the water may be too hot for a safe shower, but it would work very well to wash clothes. With a "Y" and a length of hose to a water spigot, you could mix the hot water with cold to get a cooler (but longer) shower.

Lessons Learned:

This is a good introduction to thermodynamics, even if you don't mention the term. This project shows that heat can flow just like water. You can get the heat to rise. I like this project because it is pretty much foolproof, but free experimentation and a little knowledge allows it to be tweaked for better efficiencies. A young scientist or experimenter can keep records of daily temperatures, time in the sun, layouts of the hose, and starting and final water temperatures to really begin to learn about solar heating.

PROJECT 43

HOMEMADE CHEESE CRACKERS

At my house we go through boxes upon boxes of cheese crackers. My three-year-old loves them, and while he will share if forced, he doles them out to his daddy one at a time.

When I came upon a recipe for homemade cheese crackers, as soon as I got past the excitement, I realized that this simple recipe was something that I should have been able to figure out on my own.

This is a good recipe for young cooks, as it is easy, but due to the novelty, it will get them lots of compliments from those that they share with.

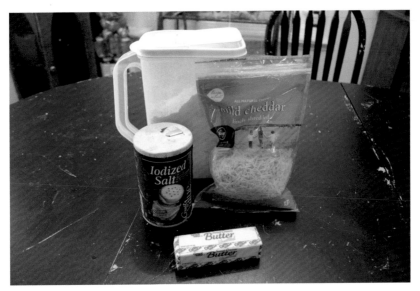

The Ingredients

Ingredients:

- 1 cup all-purpose flour
- 4 tablespoons unsalted butter, cut into small pieces
- 8 ounces sharp cheddar cheese, grated
- ¾ teaspoon salt
- 2 tablespoons cold water
- ½ teaspoon ground mustard (optional)

Tools:

- Food Processor
- Measuring cups and spoons
- Plastic wrap
- Pizza cutter
- Toothpick
- Baking sheet
- Parchment paper

Procedure:

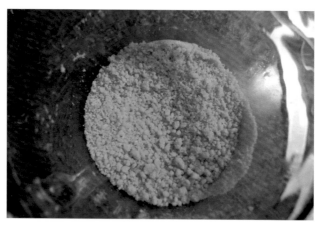

Mix until ingredients look like crumbs

1. In a food processor, pulse all the ingredients (except the water) until it looks like coarse crumbs.
2. Once you get the crumbly texture, add in water 1 tablespoon at a time while continuing to pulse the food processor.
3. Remove the mixture from the food processor

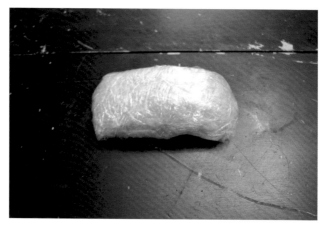

Wrap in plastic and chill

4. Wrap the mix in plastic wrap and refrigerate for at least 20 minutes.

5. Preheat oven to 350 degrees.

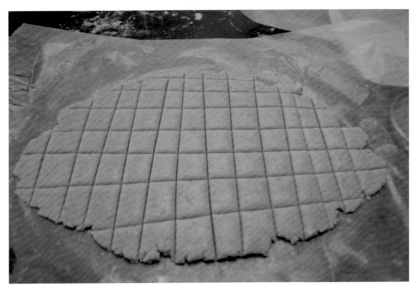

Roll thin and cut into squares

6. Roll out dough until it is very thin, and then cut into squares using a pizza cutter.

7. Use a toothpick to poke a hole in the middle of each cracker.

8. Place crackers on lined baking sheet. Since the crackers don't expand much you can put them close together.

9. Bake for 13–15 minutes or until crispy.

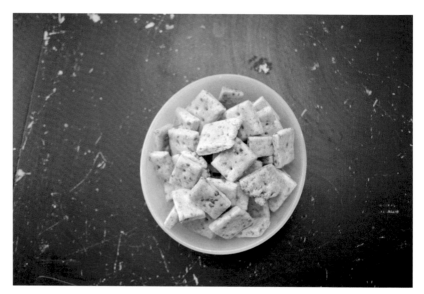

The first bake may not have the
same texture as commercial crackers,
but they are addictive

Lessons Learned:

This would be a good time to have a discussion about how things are made. Looking at how simple this recipe is, what other things from the grocery can be figured out and replicated?

PROJECT 44

MINI CAN STOVE

Material:
- Denatured alcohol
- A piece of wood
- Bottle
- 2 empty aluminum cans
- Fiberglass insulation
- Sand paper (optional)

Tools:
- Knife
- Scissors
- Small finish nail
- Hammer
- Lighter

Procedure:

1. Put the knife on your piece of wood, and make the blade touch the can with a slight pressure. Turn the can at least one complete revolution against the knife to score it.
2. Stick the scissors through the can above the score line, angle downwards, and cut the can in half along the score line.
3. Repeat step 1 and 2 on the other can.
4. Cut a notch in the bottom of one of the cans and cut it half way down the can and about ¼ inch wide. Bend it down into the inside of the can.
5. Fill up the notched can with fiberglass insulation.
6. Press the can without the notch onto the can with the fiberglass. Make a snug fit because this should not come apart.
7. Use the nail and hammer and put 4 or 5 small holes in the top of the stove (which is the "bottom" of the can without the notch and insulation) out the holes in the center of the can.
8. Put 8 more holes around the lip of the can.
9. Fill the stove with alcohol by pouring alcohol into the top slowly and allow it to soak into the fiberglass. This will take a while the first time
10. To light it, you will have to warm the alcohol up to get it to vaporize. One way is to use a tea light candle, but you could pour a small amount of alcohol on the ground around the stove (but I think that defeats the purpose).
11. To extinguish, smother the flames with a metal bowl or cup.

This is not the same as the slightly more complicated penny stove that backpackers use. This project is simpler as a introduction to metalwork.

If this is something that is interesting to you, other tin can stoves, ultra-light camping gear, or tin can metal work projects are easily found online.

Remember that cut ends of aluminum cans are very sharp. Go slow and be careful.

Lesson Learned:

Tin can metalworking is very accessible and is commonly used as an introduction to metal work.

PROJECT 45

PLASTIC BAG ICE CREAM INSERT

This is a fun way to both spend time with your family, enjoy a nice summer treat, and experiment with cold in a fun way.

Just be sure to double bag the milk and ensure everything is closed nice and tight.

Each recipe makes a single serving—you can eat it straight from the bag.

Ingredients:
- ½ cup milk
- ½ teaspoon vanilla
- 1 tablespoon sugar
- 4 cups crushed ice
- 4 tablespoons salt

Tools:
- 2 quart size freezer bags
- 1 gallon size freezer bag

- Hand towel or gloves
- Tape (optional)

Procedure:

1. Mix the milk, vanilla, and sugar together in one of the quart size bags.
2. Seal tightly, removing as much air as possible. Too much air will force the bag open during shaking.
3. Double bag the ingredient bag into the second quart bag. I like to put the top of the inner bag at the bottom of the second to minimize leaking.
4. Put the double-bagged milk mix inside the gallon size bag.
5. Fill the large bag with ice, then sprinkle salt on top.
6. Again, let all the air escape and seal the ice bag.
7. Wrap the bag in the towel or put your gloves on, and shake and massage the bag, making sure the ice surrounds the cream mixture.
8. If you tape the towel tightly around the bag you can toss it like a ball if you are not TOO rough . . .
9. Five to eight minutes is adequate time for the mixture to freeze into ice cream.

Lessons Learned:

When salt contacts ice, the freezing point of the ice is lowered.

Regular water will normally freeze at 32 degrees F. A 10% salt solution will freeze at 20 degrees F, and a 20% solution freezes at 2 degrees F.

By lowering the freezing temperature, an environment is created where the milk mix can freeze at a temperature below 32 degrees F.

PROJECT 46

PLASTIC BAG WATER COLLECTION

As a child I used to read about solar stills made by digging a hole in the desert and covering it with clear plastic. I was an adult by the time I actually visited a desert environment, but I was very disappointed with the results.

However, by placing a plastic bag over the leaves of a living plant, I was able to collect much more water in a much easier manner.

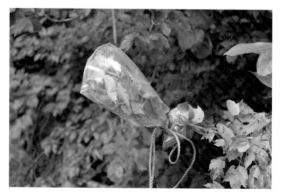

It's simple and it works

Plastic Bag Water Collection

Material:
- Several large, clear plastic bags
- String or cord
- Live, non-poisonous vegetation with green deciduous leaves

Procedure:
1. Tie a clear plastic bag on the end of a plant or small tree branch. The bag should be sealed very tightly over the branch so water cannot escape.
2. Water vapor will collect and condense in the bag.
3. Wait until evening for maximum condensation before removing the bag.
4. Switch the bag to another branch and repeat.

Yield:
You can expect an average of one cup of water per bag per day—which means you will need 16 of these devices per person to collect the minimum recommended one gallon per person per day of water.

Lessons Learned:
This project can lead to discussions about survival efficiencies—the need to try a skill rather than just trusting in techniques you have read about. It also illustrates the difference in deciduous and evergreen trees. Deciduous trees shed their leaves during the winter because water is at a premium and most of the water a tree root absorbs is lost through the leaves.

PROJECT 47

POPSICLE STICK LOOM

Weaving is one of the most ancient technologies. The machines used to help us weave are called looms. Unfortunately, most looms cost hundred or thousands of dollars.

Today we are going to make a small loom out of Popsicle sticks. This loom is the perfect size to make things like potholders and hanging decorations.

While the type of loom we are going to make makes small cloth squares, in many places, South Africa for instance, the squares are sewn together to make very beautiful clothing.

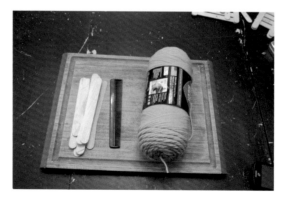

The Materials

Material:

- 12 Popsicle sticks
- Wide and thin piece of wood to make a "shuttle"
- Yarn

Tools:

- Glue
- Drill with small bit.
- Hair comb
- Table

Procedure:

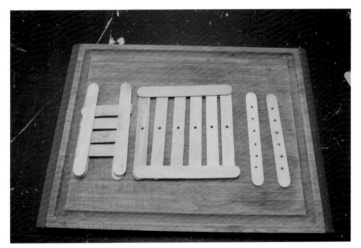

Competed loom parts (Left to right: Shuttle, Heddle, and the two spreaders)

1. Drill a small hole in the center of 6 of the Popsicle sticks.
2. Lay the 6 sticks out equally and connect them by gluing sticks to the top and bottom of the 6 sticks to make a "ladder" shape. This makes the "Heddle."

3. Drill 6 small holes equally spaced down the center of two more Popsicle sticks.

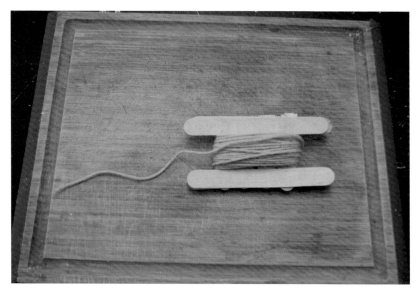

Yarn on shuttle

4. Construct the shuttle by wrapping a good amount of thread around a narrow piece of wood or ridged plastic—it needs to have a lot of thread, but not so bulky it can't fit between the threads on the loom.

Setup:

1. Cut a piece of yarn into six pieces, each 3 to 4 feet long.
2. Find the center of each piece and double it over.
3. Tie the 6 yarn sections together at the looped over center portion. This should make a bundle of looped yarn at one end, and 12 free ends.
4. Tie the looped end to a table or tree—something you can pull against.

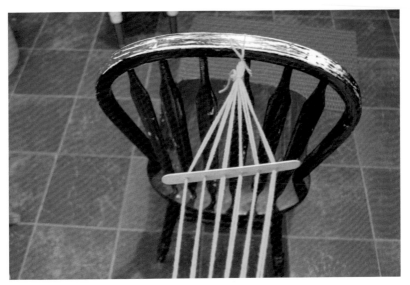

Yarn through spreader and anchored on chair

5. Take two of the free ends of the yarn bundle and push them both through the leftmost hole in one of the Popsicle sticks with 6 holes.

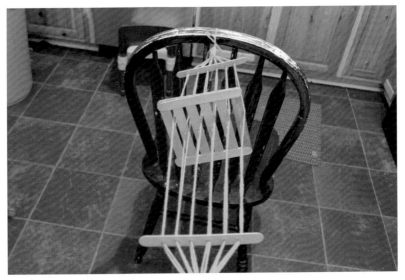

Front view of heddle on yarn

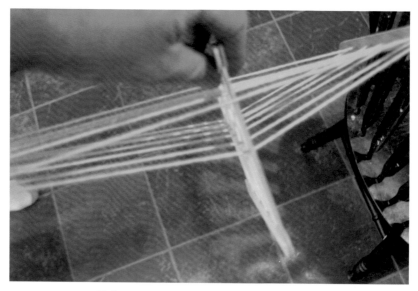

Side view of heddle on yarn

6. Now that two pieces of yarn are stuck through one hole in the end stick, take one of those yarn pieces and push it through the hole in the leftmost stick of the heddle. Then take the second yarn end and push it through the heddle between the leftmost heddle stick and the next one.

7. Gather both pieces of yarn and push them through the leftmost hole of the second Popsicle stick with 6 holes.

8. Repeat steps 5–7 with two more yarn sections, and using the next set of holes.

9. Do this until all 6 holes in the end sticks are filled, and the heddle has a single string through each hole, and a piece of yarn between each set of uprights.

10. Gather the loose ends of yarn as they pass through the 6 holed spreader stick; tie them together.

11. Tie the mass of yarn to your belt.

12. Tie the end of the yarn on your shuttle to the thread on the far left of your loom.

Weaving:

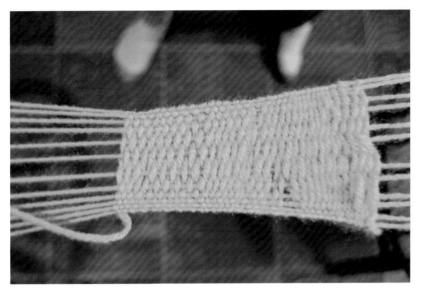

Weaving

1. Back up from the stationary end so the threads are tight.
2. Ensure that all the threads are of equal length.
3. Lift your heddle up with one hand to make a triangle of threads in the heddle. (When lifting or depressing the heddle, only the threads in the hole will move. The threads between the sticks will always stay in line with the two end sticks.)
4. Push your shuttle through this triangle, pulling it back toward you to tighten the thread.
5. Drop the heddle down, making a triangle of yarn in the other direction.
6. Pass the shuttle through the triangle, tightening it as you go.
7. Lift the heddle and pass the shuttle through.

8. Keep alternating the heddle up and down, and passing the shuttle through until you have woven the cloth the size you desire.

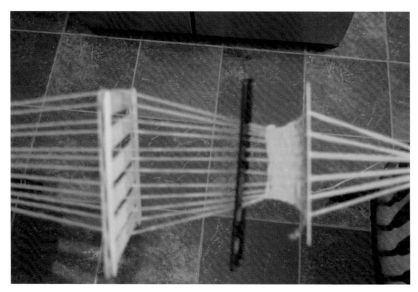

Use comb to keep weave tight

9. Between weaves, use a comb to pull the threads toward you to keep the weave tight.
10. When done, cut the yarn from the sticks, pull out the heddle, and tie the strings on each end together.

Lessons Learned:

This neat craft project is an example of experimental anthropology—it shows how our ancestors made cloth thousands of years ago. It shows how things are made, and fosters appreciation of the items we take for granted.

PROJECT 48

FISHING BUTTON

I first saw this on a Doomsday Prepper video from Scott Hunt, but I have also seen it many other places online. After making some modifications of my own, I decided to make a couple to stick in my bug out bags. It is smaller and lighter than the other PVC fishing pole used in project 26, and much more efficient to use than the sinkers in project 37's survival kit—which places it straight in the middle of your options.

Depending on how much you like to fish, how good you are at it, and how likely it is that you will encounter areas where you may end up fishing while out exploring, you may want to keep one or more of the three options available to you.

As I have said online, in print, and in person, I think PVC is one of the DIYer's best materials, and anyone with a little imagination can use this inexpensive material to solve all manner of problems them may have.

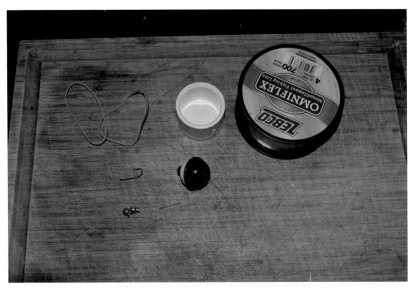

The Materials

Material:

- Small plastic fishing bobber
- PVC end cap—size needed is determined by the size of your bobber. The easiest thing to do is to buy a bobber and take it with you to the hardware store and match it up.
- Small fishing hook
- Lead split shot sinker
- Fishing line
- Small washer
- Rubber band

Tools:

- Hacksaw blade
- File
- Small drill bit and drill

Procedure:

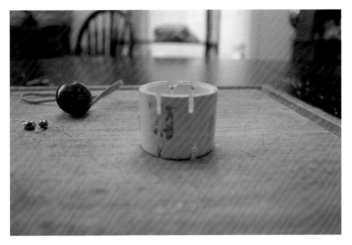

Make cuts

1. Cut two slots ¼ inch deep and about ⅓ inch apart on the bottom end of the PVC Cap.
2. Turn the cap on its side and carefully saw the plastic to connect the slots cut into the PVC cap.

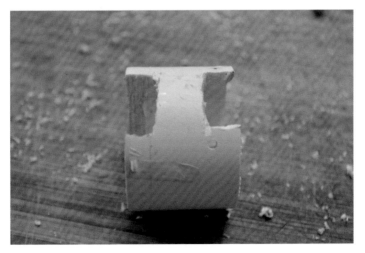

Connect cuts

3. Once the connecting cut is deep enough, snap the square of plastic between the two slots off of the PVC end cap.
4. Flip the cap over and repeat steps 2 and 3 on the other side of the cap.
5. Using a file, carefully clean out the two notches made on the bottom end of the cap.
6. Set the cap down on a firm work area and carefully cut two more parallel slots ¼ inch deep, and ⅓ inch apart across the top of the PVC cap.
7. The cuts on the top of the cap should be in line with the cuts you made on the bottom—It should look like an "H."
8. Connect the slots by cutting into the side of the cap just as you did in step 2.
9. Snap off the plastic between the two slots—it may be harder on the top than the bottom, but have patience.
10. Clean out the notches with a file, just as you did on step 5.
11. Take a small drill bit, and drill a hole about ⅛ inch away from the bottom corner of one of the notches you made.
12. Tie a small hook to a length of fishing line, and add a couple of lead sinkers near the hook.
13. Thread the line through the hole drilled into the PVC cap.
14. Tie the washer to the other end of the fishing line.

To Pack:

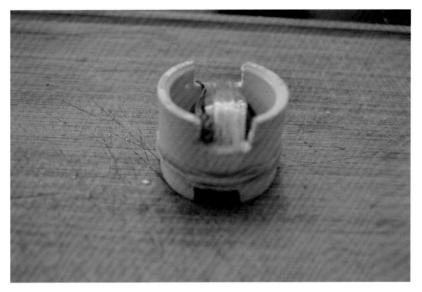

Assemble

1. Insert the bobber into the center of the PVC cap.
2. Place the hook on the outside of the cap, and pull the barbed end of the hook down and into the notch cut into the cap—this keeps it from getting loose and sticking you.
3. Pull the washer end of the fishing line through the hole, which will tend to lock the hook into the cap.
4. Wrap the line around the notches until all the line is secure.
5. Stick the washer between the loops of fishing line and the side of the cap.
6. Wrap a rubber band around the fishing line to keep it from unraveling.

To Use:

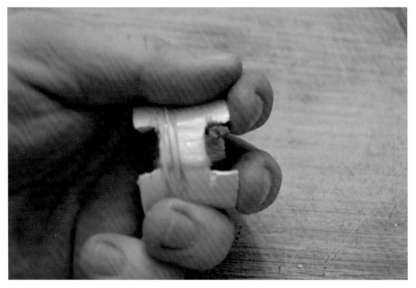

Hold line between fingers with
button in your palm

1. Remove rubber band.
2. Unwrap line.
3. Remove bobber
4. Pull fishing hook out and pull line until the washer is pulled up into the PCV cap.
5. Wrap line around endcap, leaving enough line free to cast.
6. Attach bobber and bait hook.
7. Hold cap in the palm of your non-dominant hand and let string out between your index and middle fingers, wrapping the rest of your fingers into a fist.
8. Hold the baited end in your dominant hand, swinging the hook in circles.
9. Cast the hook, by aiming and releasing the swinging hook in the direction you wish to fish.

10. When a fish bites—set the hook by holding the cap firmly, and pulling back sharply on the line.
11. Enjoy your fish.

Lesson Learned:

This project reinforces creativity, and finding novel uses for common materials. As the last fishing project, it also sets up a perfect time for a fishing trip to experiment and compare the three fishing set ups made in this book.

PROJECT 49

FIRST AID KIT

You can't really be prepared without owning a first aid kit. Even someone that does not self-identify as a "prepper" should have a first aid kit.

If you do not want to buy a ready built kit—either to save money, or to ensure you have quality materials tailored to your use, this project helps you create your own.

The materials listed are not exhaustive, and are just common items found in good kits. Feel free to substitute items or add to this list.

Material:
- 2 absorbent compress dressings (5 x 9 inches)
- 25 adhesive bandages (assorted sizes)
- 1 adhesive cloth tape (10 yards x 1 inch)
- package of moleskin for blisters.
- 5 antibiotic ointment packets (approximately 1 gram)
- 5 antiseptic wipe packets
- 2 packets of aspirin (81 mg each)

First Aid Kit

- 1 blanket (space blanket)
- 1 breathing barrier (with one-way valve)
- 1 instant cold compress
- 2 pair of non-latex gloves (size: large)
- 2 hydrocortisone ointment packets (approximately 1 gram each)
- Scissors
- 1 roller bandage (3 inches wide)
- 1 roller bandage (4 inches wide)
- 5 sterile gauze pads (3 x 3 inches)
- 5 sterile gauze pads (4 x 4 inches)
- Oral thermometer (non-mercury/non-glass)
- Small penlight or flashlight.
- 2 triangular bandages
- Tweezers
- First aid instruction booklet
- Index card
- Pen
- Personal prescriptions as appropriate
- Small bag

Procedure:

1. When packing emergency kits, I like to keep non-emergency, but commonly used items in outside pockets. Consider doing this with things like aspirin, ointments, and Band-Aids.
2. Try to keep items used less commonly on the bottom of the pack to free room to store any emergency items like the breathing barrier and large bandages on top for quick access.

3. Use the index card and pen to write any emergency phone numbers and instructions (like medical alert information)
4. Check the kit regularly to ensure the flashlight works and nothing has been removed, contaminated, or expired.

Lessons Learned:

This kit gives the opportunity to discuss age appropriate emergency procedures. For young children it may be when (and when not) to dial 911. Older children may be ready for first aid instruction or actual certification courses.

By building this kit after you are familiar with the Doctor Game in project 33, you can have a fun discussion of what common items can be used to replace the items found in the kit. Examples would be duct tape for the moleskin or a bandanna for the triangular bandage.

PROJECT 50

BURNED BOWL

One of my more vivid childhood memories is sitting around a campfire with my dad as I made a burned out bowl using coals.

Not only is this a fun way to make a useful item, this technique has been used by Native Americans to build much larger items like log canoes without the use of any tools.

It is very simple to do, and doesn't take much time, but as with any fire project, you need to take care not get burned, and ensure you have some means to extinguish fire close at hand.

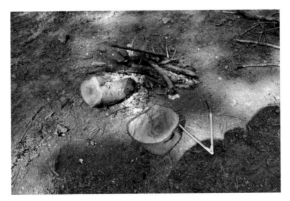

The Material

Material:

- Small or medium sized piece of solid wood
- Campfire
- Boiled linseed oil or vegetable oil

Tools:

- Metal tongs, or a green limb trimmed in the middle and bent into tongs
- Metal spoon, sharp rock or other scraper
- Fire extinguisher, water hose, or bucket of sand
- Knife
- Straw (Optional)
- Sandpaper
- Rag

Procedure:

1. Light a campfire and let it burn to coals.
2. If you don't have a set of metal tongs, make one by finding a straight length of green branch about 2 feet long and as big around as an adult thumb. Make sure this is from a non-poisonous hardwood tree like oak.
3. Trim off any small side branches, and carefully scrape down a few inches of the branch in the center of the limb. By scraping down a little past halfway through the green branch, you should be able to bend it without breaking.
4. Trim the ends to make a semi-flat end to enable you to use the bent branch as tongs to pick up small rocks. Don't cut too much or the hot coals may burn through.

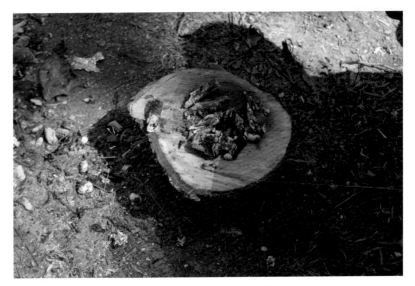

Set coals on your bowl

5. Once the fire is burned to hot coals, and your tongs are ready, use them to pick up a couple coals and place them on the center of the wood you want to burn out.

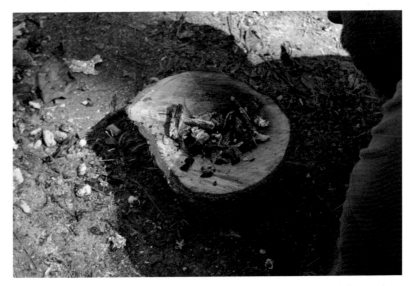

Blow to cause coals to burn out your bowl

6. Blow gently on the coal where it meets the wood. A straw may help direct the air. The idea is to carefully burn small areas of the wood in a controlled area.
7. Once the wood chars a little, dump out the coal and scrape out the charred area.

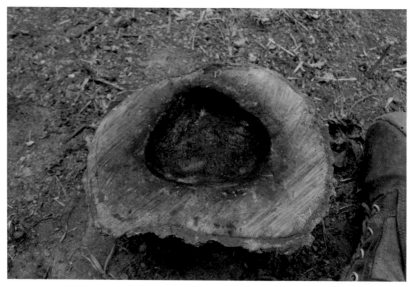

Gouge out charred wood and add coals until bowl is deep as you desire

8. By strategic use of the coals, air, and scraping, a depression can be burned out of the log.
9. Once the log is burned deep enough to make a bowl that satisfies, scrape it out completely, and sand it until you are happy with both the inner bowl and outer wood.
10. Once sanded, pour oil onto the bowl and rub it in with the rag.* It may take several coats and a couple days, but eventually the oil will soak in and harden and make a very pretty and useful bowl.

*Oils and natural rag fibers can become hazardous. As the oil oxidizes in the rag it will make heat. Many shops have burned when the heat ignites the rag. I always burn my rags after using them with oil.

Lessons Learned:

This project teaches the confidence of mastering fire—It shows that with knowledge and care dangerous things can be mastered and turned into tools.

It is also a primal outlet for creativity and artistry. These bowls are useful, but they can be beautiful and valuable works of art.

It also can be used to grow appreciation for modern items like plastic bowls.

PROJECT 51

WHIPPING ROPE AND TYING KNOTS

Being able to use rope efficiently is more than an old-time pioneer skill. Proper knots are distinguished by their ability to hold when needed, release easily when needed, and not reduce the strength of the rope any more than required.

While everyone can tie "granny" knots and bend rope around, the ability to know and use the right knot for the right use is a pleasure and is a testament to skill and professionalism.

In this project we will show how to prevent rope ends from unraveling by whipping the ends, as well as prepare for the last project in the book by showing how to tie some common knots. They are:

- Square knot
- Clove Hitch
- Tautline Hitch
- Bowline

While there are hundreds of specialty knots, I find I can do most every common task with just these four knots.

While not as common, we will also show a timber hitch as it is used in diagonal lashing.

Before we get into the knots, let's prepare our practice rope by whipping the ends so that they do not unravel.

Material:
- Rope
- Thread

Tools:
- Knife

Procedure:
1. Loop the end of a 2 foot piece of thread, string, or twine—in knot tying terms, a loop is called a bight.
    1.1. One end of the bight should be just a little longer than the distance you want to whip, so that the majority of your string is on the other end of the bight.
2. Lay your bight against the end of the rope you wish to whip, and the bight should be parallel to the rope.
3. While holding the bight against the rope, and starting near the end of the short end of your string loop, take the long end of string and wrap it around the rope.
4. Keep the wrap tight and continue to wrap the string neatly until the wraps are roughly equal to the diameter of the rope you are whipping.

5. Reeve the end of the twine through the eye of the bight. This means thread the loose end of the twine you are wrapping through the loop sticking out from your wraps.
6. Pull on the end of the twine that is extending beyond the end of the rope until the bight at the free end of the twine is pulled under and to the mid point of the wrappings.
7. Finish the whipping by cutting off the ends of the twine.

Now for the knots. . . .

Square Knot

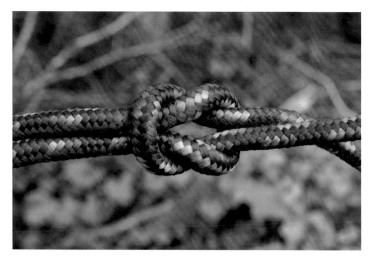

Square Knot

The square knot is probably the best known knot. It is easy to tie and is useful for low strain ties.

The knot is popular among sailors, climbers, and gift wrappers for its convenience and ease of tying.

One of the simplest knots available, the square knot nevertheless proves plenty strong for most casual applications.

What I like best about it is that if you grab one rope ends that are not under strain, and pull it back toward the knot, a properly tied square knot will untie itself. Unfortunately, this makes it unreliable for climbing.

Tying the Square Knot:
1. Take two ropes and lay the right-hand rope over the other.
2. Wrap the right-hand rope under the left-hand rope.
3. Bring the right-hand rope back over the left-hand rope.
4. Bring the original right-hand rope over the other rope.
5. Pull the original right-hand rope under the other rope.
6. Pull on both ends firmly to tighten.

Clove Hitch

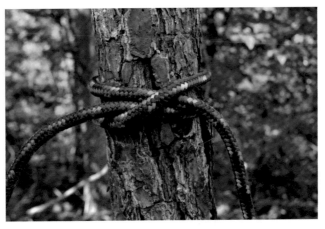

Clove Hitch

A clove hitch is used to tie a rope to a cylindrical object (like a fence post or tree), this makes it essential for lashing (tying timbers together to build useful items), but be aware that it is unreliable when tied on a square post.

It is also useful to know that that if you feed the rope in from either end the knot will loosen—making it adjustable.

Basically it is just two half-hitches tied in a row

Tying the Clove Hitch:

1. To tie a clove hitch at the end of a rope, pass the end around the pole starting at the right, with the end coming around below.
2. Put the end around in the same direction to cross over the standing end to be above the first loop.
3. As the end comes around, put it under itself to be over the standing end.
4. Check that both ends are in the middle, emerging in opposite directions.
5. Pull to tighten.

When pulled tighter, the rope passing over itself binds it in place.

Tautline Hitch

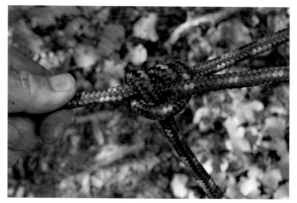

Tautline Hitch

Since it can be slipped to tighten or loosen a line, and it also holds well under load, the tautline hitch is a great knot for camping.

This knot is most often used to attach lines to tents and tarps, but it is also used on occasion to tie down loads on trailers.

Tying the Tautline Hitch:

1. Make a turn around a post or other object several feet from the free end.
2. Coil the free end twice around the standing line working back toward the post.
3. Make one additional coil around the standing line on the outside of the coils just made.
4. Tighten the knot and slide it on the standing line to adjust tension.

Bowline

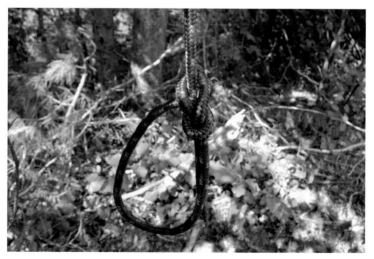

Bowline

Anytime you tie a knot in a rope you reduce its strength through bending; the better the knot, the less strength you lose, and a properly tied bowline retains about 65 percent of its strength.

Because a bowline retains a good bit of the rope's natural strength, the Federal Aircraft Administration uses it to tie down light aircraft. More importantly, the bowline is commonly used as a rescue knot for conscious individuals that fell into holes or off cliffs. I even have a video on my YouTube channel that shows how a person can tie a bowline with one hand in the event they are injured and have a rope thrown down to them.

Tying the Bowline:
1. Lay the rope across your left hand with the free end hanging down.
2. Form a small loop in the line in your hand.
3. Bring the free end up to and pass through the eye from the under side.
4. Wrap the line around the standing line and back down through the loop.
5. Tighten the knot by pulling on free end while holding standing line.

Timber Hitch

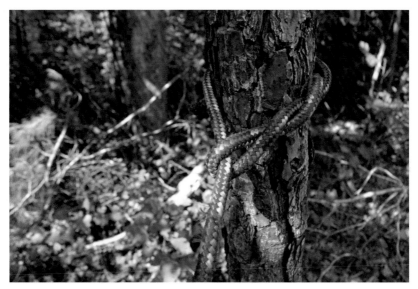

Timber Hitch

The timber hitch is used to secure a rope around a post or any cylindrical object. It does not jam or slip, no matter how heavy the load, and is easy to tie and untie.

Tying the Timber Hitch:

1. Pass the working end of a rope around the object and take a turn around the standing part.
2. Tuck the working end back around itself three times with the lay of the rope.
3. Add one or two half hitches near the hauling end for hoisting and to keep load from twisting.

Lessons Learned:

This particular project is of lifetime use. I learned knots as a preteen, and use them all the time. It is nice to know how to use the proper tool for the right use. This project provides a good time to discuss why using proper techniques is important, and that it is okay to have pride in doing a job the right way.

PROJECT 52

LASHING

Lashing is the process of connecting timbers together to build things. I use lashing all the time when camping or while out on the farm.

You can use lashing to build bridges, benches, tables, towers, fences, and tent frames. Even buildings can be made with lashing.

This is a great tool for the creative because with a little rope, some poles, and some skill you can form just about anything.

Here are the main types of lashing we will use:
- Square lashing is used to bind spars together.
- Diagonal lashing is used to bind poles together.
- Shear lashing is used for lashing together two parallel spars, which will be opened out of the parallel to form sheer legs as in the formation of an A-frame.

Before we begin, you should become familiar with some commonly used terms when describing the lashing.

Spars: Poles to be lashed together.

Wrap: A series of turns of cordage around two or more spars (poles) you're binding together.

Frap: Turns of cordage on top and perpendicular to the previous wraps. Fraps go between the spars to pull the joint tight.

Tag End: The short end of your cordage when tying knots and lashings.

Working End: The long end of your cordage when tying knots and lashings.

Material:
- Rope/Twine (diameter and strength should be tied to the size of the poles and what you wish to make)
- Poles (length and size depends on what you wish to make)

Tools:
- Knife

Types of Lashing:
Square lashing

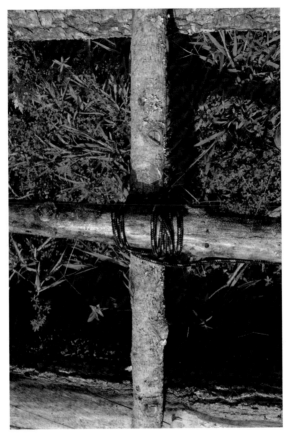

Square Lashing

1. Tie a clove hitch on the bottom pole right next to the intersecting pole.
2. After the clove hitch, make 3 tight wraps around both poles.
   o Wrap the rope in and out in between the poles.
   o The wraps should be collecting on the pole going sideways.

3. Put two fraps in between both poles in the opposite direction of the wraps.
   o Make sure you do the wraps and fraps tight or else it will be weak.
4. After making sure everything is taut, tie another clove hitch on the top pole.
5. Cut off the excess rope on the end.

Diagonal lashing

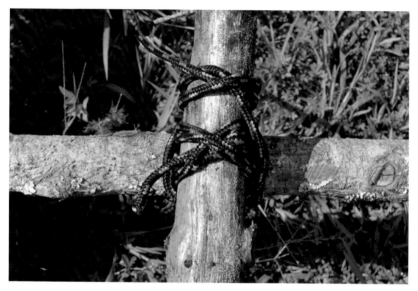

Diagonal Lashing

1. Cinch the poles together by tying a Timber Hitch around them where they cross.
2. Make three to four wrapping turns on the opposite diagonal to the Timber Hitch.
   o Keep the wraps parallel to one another and pull them tight.

3. Make three more tight wraps across the first three, again keeping them parallel.
4. Take two to three frapping turns between the poles, tightly around both sets of wraps
5. Complete the lashing with a Clove Hitch around one of the poles.

Shear Lashing

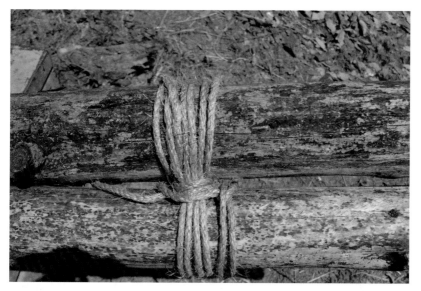

Shear Lashing

1. Lay two spars side by side.
2. Tie a clove hitch to one spar.
3. Make four loose wraps around the spars.
4. Make four frapping turns between the spars.
5. Finish with a clove hitch.

Things to make with Lashing:

- Two long poles lashed parallel to each other using square lashing to two trees, and covered with smaller sticks makes a great camp table.
- Diagonal lashing can make trestles for a rope bridge.
- See if you can lash together a larger heddle to weave things much bigger than the popsicle loom you made earlier.

Experiment with your lashings to make anything you want.

About the Author

David is the father of William Tell, a very precocious little toddler. W. T.'s parents spend long hours working with him to ensure that he grows up to be an independent and hardworking adult who is not afraid to follow his dreams.

When not engaged in peekaboo, playing in the sprinkler, or locked in life or death foam sword battles, David is a full time Emergency Manager, Author, and Instructor.

You can find him online at www.tngun.com